My Adventures into Food Medicine

Joseph Cheroong Cho

조 가 양 생 비 법

인류를 근원적으로 질병과
고통으로부터 해방시키는
누구나 선택할 수 있는
필수불가결의 자연 건강법

"미끈미끈/끈적끈적"한 성질을 가진 식물섬유질의
간단없는 섭취가 열쇠라. 소변에 풍성한 거품있죠?
그것이 질병을 씻어내는 눈에 보이는 증거올시다.
이 거품이 식도에 머물러 있을 때 물을 마시면 씻
겨내려가 위장에 도달함으로써 무기물질인 천연수
를 유기화함으로써 질병이 예방되는 비결로 보임.
섬유질 섭취를 평생 계속하면 평생무병장수떼놓은
당상이요! 이것은 자연의 약속이요, 자연은 속이지
아니하며, 아무도 자연을 속일 수도 없습니다. 이
섬유소를 풍성하게 함유하는 식품들의 몇가지 예:
**열무김치, 총각김치, 겨울철 그늘에 말린 무 씨레기, 쪄서 말린
고구마 줄거리, 등등…뿐만
아니라, 마, 다시마, 미역 등 모든 해초나물, 모든 식물류나물,
집 마당가에 키운 Okra 등등.**

CONTENTS

PROFESSIONAL EXPERIENCES

- Born on Dec. 15, 1940 in South Korea. Translated from English and got published SEEDS OF CONTEMPLATION BY THOMAS MERTON ~ 명상의 씨~ by Catholic Public Company in Korea in July 1961.

- From January 1964 through December 31, 1966 I was employed as an editorial assistant for the City and Country (Monthly) Magazine of the Catholic Church, publication section, through Dec. 31 1966.

- From January 1967 through June 1973 (for about 6 and half years) I was selected the first place out of 900+ applicants, with a few others, in a set of written exams to be formally trained to be a professional newspaper reporter by Kyunghyang Shinmoon Daily Newspaper in Korea for 18 months, and then worked for the company mostly as political reporter, 6 full days every week. I wrote several feature stories assigned by editors for the newspaper in addition to the daily reporting duties. Visited a few Southeast Asian countries with some fellow reporters reporting the activities of the visiting Korean Foreign Minister.

- In July 1973 I came to Chicago to visit a friend and eventually enrolled in the graduate school of the University of Illinois at Urbana-Champaign, Illinois and was awarded a Master's Degree in Advertising in January 1976.

- Upon Completion of 18 quarters of graduate studies during 4 and half years, 1995 through June 1999, all required courses of Oriental Medicine at Samra University of Oriental Medicine, I received Master of Science in Oriental Medicine (MSOM) degree on June 30, 1999.

- Upon satisfactory completion of all requirements, I was awarded Acupuncture Licensure to practice acupuncture in the State of California, on January 25, 2000, and subsequently opened an office in Glendale, California, which I called Yang Saeng Dang, through February 2006, and moved to Black Mountain, North Carolina.

I HAVE SUFFERED FROM SINUS TROUBLES FOR NEARLY 50 YEARS SINCE AGE 30, WHEN I MOVED TO CHICAGO AND WAS EXPOSED TO THE FREEZING TEMPERATURE, CHILLY WINDS

FROM THE LAKE MICHIGAN, AND THE RAGWEED BLOOMS IN THE WARMER SEASONS, OR WHAT HAVE YOU, AND I WAS ON MEDICATION EVER SINCE.

BESIDES, I HAD A THEORY THAT THE HUMANITY SHOULD HAVE HAD A NATURAL HEALTH PROTECTION FROM THE VERY, VERY EARLY BEGINNING OF THEIR LIFE ON EARTH THROUGH SOME KIND OF FIRM PROTECTION BY THE MOTHER NATURE, AND WITHOUT WHICH THE HUMANIY COULD'NT POSSIBLY HAVE SURVIVED THESE THOUSANDS OF SHEAVES OF YEARS. AND I FURTHER THEORIZED THAT OUR TRIBAL ANCESTORS LIVING IN DIFFERENT REGIONS THROUGHOUT THE WORLD ESTABLISHED THEIR OWN DIET PROTECING THEIR HEALTH AND THE PROSPERITY OF THEIR OWN TRIBES, AND TAUGHT THEIR CHILDREN TO STICK TO IT. AND THAT'S HOW HUMANITY SURVIVED THOUSANDS AND THOUSANDS OF YEARS UNTIL TODAY, I BELIEVED.

PARTLY TIRED OF MY LONG DEPENDENCE ON MEDICATION, AND PARTLY MOTIVATED FROM MY DESIRE TO PROVE MY THEORY OF NATURAL PROTECTION, I QUIT THE MEDICATION COLD TURKEY AND USHERED IN MY FOOD-ONLY HEALING EXPERIMENT IN MARCH 2012, WHEN I HAD TEMORARILY MOVED BACK TO KOREA TO CARE FOR MY AGING MOTHER AND 6-7-8 YEARS LATER I AM CLEAR OF ANY SINUS SYMPTOMS NOW, AND HOPEFULLY FREE FROM ANY DISEASE WHATSOEVER, AS LONG AS I MAY LIVE, AT THE MOTHER NATURE'S GRACE.

I MOVED BACK AND FORTH A LITTLE BIT, FROM SOUTHERN CALIFORNIA TO NORTH CAROLINA. I LOVED MOUNTAIN HIKING THERE AND GOT MY BIG TOE MISHAP THERE ON THE NOVEMBER FIRST, WITH THE FIRST SNOW FLURIES THERE. MY YOUNGER BROTHER HAD A PROBLEM WITH OUR AGING MOM IN KOREA, SO I HAD TO MOVE BACK TO KOREA, AND FOUND A HOME TO SETTLE DOWN WITH MY MOM IN GOSUNG, SOUTH KOREA, IN FEBRUARY 2012. IN A COUPLE OF YEARS, THINGS GOT SMOOTHED OUT AND OUR AGING

MOTHER WAS HAPPY TO MOVE BACK WITH HER YOUNGER SON AND DAUGHER-IN-LAW. I TELL YOU, MY READERS, THAT ACTUALLY I STARTED "MY NO MEDICINE BUT FOOD ONLY EXPERIMENT," WHILE I STARTED LIVING WITH, AND CARING MY MOM IN FEBRUARY, 2012.

THIS IS MY PERSONAL FACTUAL REPORT. YOU CAN EASILY REPLICATE MY EXPERIENCE AND PROVE IT TO YOURSELF. I ENCOURAGE YOU, AND CHALLENGE YOU PLEASE DO SO. THE RECENT 2020 DEMOCRATIC ELECTION CAMPAIGN IN THE UNITED STATES REVEALED THAT MOST PEOPLE SEEMED TO DEMAND HEALTHCARE FROM THE GOVERNMENT OF THE UNITED STATES. LET THEM KNOW THE TRUE LIFETIME HEALTH PROTECTION BY MOTHER NATURE IS AVAILABLE RIGHT HERE AND NOW FOR THEM, FOR EVERYBODY, REGARDLESS RICH OR POOR! *THIS INFORMATION WOULD BE A GREAT EQUALIZER FOR OUR SOCIETY.* IT JUST NEEDS SOME LEAD TIME AS IT TOOK ME 6-7-8 YEARS TO BE COMPLETELY HEALED OF MY 50 YEARS LONG CHRONIC DISEASE. SO GO AHEAD REPLICATE MY SUCCESS AND CHANCES ARE THAT YOU WILL MOST LIKELY BE COMPLETELY FREE OF ANY EXISTING ORGANIC DISEASE AND PAIN DUE TO THE DISEASE, AND AS YOU WILL CONTINUE WITH YOUR MUCILAGE RICH/ OR FIBER RICH FOOD, YOU WILL BECOME YOUR OWN BOSS ON YOUR LIFETIME PERSONAL HEALTHCARE BY MOTHER NATURE'S GRACE.

THIS IS CERTAINLY SOMETHING WORTH YOUR WHILE! KEEP YOUR MIND CLEAR AND FIRMLY INDEPENDENT, RELYING ON YOUR NATURAL PERSONAL INSTINCTUAL INTELLIGENCE YOU'RE BORN WITH. ALWAYS! THAT'S THE KEY!

AND PRACTICE PERSONAL SELF CARE, GENETICALLY HANDED DOWN IN YOUR OWN VERY PHYSICAL BODY AND PROTECTED BY MOTHER NATURE. THAT MAY GIVE

YOURSELF THE BEST HEALTHCARE THERE IS. READ ON FOR THE DETAILS!

Preface

I was walking down the street one day in Seoul, Korea, where I lived then perhaps sometime in 1967-68 or thereabout and came across an old college friend who was carrying a little box in his hand. "Hello!" I called him out and asked him where he was going. He opened the box and showed me a device that he described as a 'perpetual motion generator' he invented. He told me he was on his way to the (Korean) Patent Office. His machine could generate electricity with no fuel indefinitely, he explained. I marveled at his ingenuity and wished him luck. And I have never heard from him since. We were both young then and chasing our dreams.

"Perpetual motion is impossible theoretically as well as in reality but still a very popular pursuit," declares a website dedicated to the subject. Chasing something widely considered impossible has its romantics, I guess. Once you got hooked on, it's hard to give up, for I know from my personal experience that I'm still in the game of pursuing dreams in my 80's of years. I have been chasing something seemingly similarly impossible: a panacea, sort of. Ginseng was considered something like it in the Orient and so Carolus Linnaeus named it Panax ginseng in an allusion to its reputation. It became clear to me early enough, however, that Panax ginseng was not my kind of panacea. It was too expensive, first of all, to be widely made available to the people of moderate means, one of my top priorities. ***What I had in my mind was nothing less than something that would help lift the humanity broadly from pain and suffering due to diseases.***

I became a California Licensed Acupuncturist at age 59 and opened an office the next year in Glendale, California. I called it Yang Saeng Dang, because that was something I always was thinking about, I mean "Yang Saeng" or nurturing your life.

"Yang saeng in Korean or yang sheng in Chinese refers to the ancient Taoist tradition of nurturing life, and Dang, or Tang in Chinese, means the house. Thus Yang Saeng Dang purports to be the House of Nurturing Life in the Taoist traditions for you."

I explained in back of my business card then. Nurturing life, or cultivating for my own health through the means of diet and lifestyle, has been my undaunted passion ever since because I felt it offered a real path to the health at my control as long as I may live. The tradition also says in part,

"The good doctor treats the healthy. The one who treats the sick is only an average doctor." This needs some explaining. It means a good doctor is supposed to keep his patients healthy and from falling sick, and if your patients fall sick you are not a good doctor but just an average one. This may have been an ideal for some in an era long gone. To tell you the truth, it has become my overriding goal and ethic at the time. And still it is. Even my own son derided me, calling me "a do-gooder" and might have given up on my chances of making myself a successful practitioner ever. True, I wanted to be such a good one. To some eyes my pursuit may look foolhardy.

Was this just a pipe dream? Nobody would take me seriously. But I never gave up on my dream and was driven underground for it turned out soon that I wasn't producing enough income to help me stay in business and I had to close the Glendale office after 5 years, and never returned.

My obsession of being a good doctor, however, lingered, although I have never returned to active acupuncture and Eastern Medicine practice to date. Still, I agonized over it and wasted years beating the bushes, for I felt deeply convinced inside that an internal logic was on my side for I thought humans are product of nature, and any divergences from the natural courses, such as the degenerative diseases plaguing us today, may be corrected by returning to the primordial food that shaped us from the currently prevailing food in the modern industrialized societies. Therefore, my focus was zeroing in on the food question asking what it was the material difference between our current diet and that of early ancestors, that shaped us genetically through the primordial period, was my primary concern. So I thought I might have a chance at cracking at it.

Eventually, I had hunches here and there:

First, the legendary stories of Egyptian pharaoh's healing with jute plants, also known as, molokheia, or as Egyptian spinach, which yields *slippery and sticky stuff* when cooked in water and thus became popular as soup thickener in Egypt and her neighboring countries in the Middle East but also in an unlikely place like in Japan; I obtained the seeds of this plant, and planted in my garden, studied and used the plant for a number of years, verified and loved its *slippery and sticky stuff* as I stayed in Korea temporarily and later back to the U.S. first in Virginia, and later back to California. (Jute: the glossy fiber of either of the East Indian plants (*Corchorus olitorius* and *C. capsularis*) of the linden family used chiefly for sacking, burlap and twine. But the young plants are eaten like spinach, and are very popular in Japan, I hear. I just kept a few plants in a corner of my yard, and kept picking the fresh and tender new shoots on the mature plants, which kept coming back and were just as good and tender as of the new plants.

Second, the Native North Americans' and some of their early European settler neighbors' stories of healing again with ***slippery and sticky stuff*** from slippery elm tree's inner barks became famous and widely known; and were described in a book describing the lives of the early European pioneers settling in the North American continent among the native Americans. I took interest in finding these people living in the North America found the same ***slippery and sticky stuff*** in a totally different plant, that is, in a tree later identified as slippery elm tree. I joined a small group led by a published biologist and a farmer of Chinese medicinal plants in the State of Missouri, and the biologist identified a slippery elm tree as a medicinal, although he didn't elaborate how it was used, or for what. However, I have never used the elm tree inner bark myself and am just sharing the story with you. (Later, while I was temporarily caring for my aging Mother, I actually bought by mail 2lbs of what was purported to be the slippery elm tree bark dried and powdered from a seller in the U.S.. which failed to help anyway. But I trusted the healing stories described in the book of the European pioneers and their neighboring Native Americans.)

Third, with the thousands of years-long history of so called Yin herbs of the Traditional Chinese Medicine, or the Traditional Eastern Medicine, where something called "Yin Essence" turns out to be exactly the same stuff as referred to as ***slippery and sticky stuff*** so far.

I drew a line over the globe connecting the dots widely apart – thousands of miles across the oceans – from one another. And soon a hypothesis emerged in my head for there was an unmistakable commonality there! ***Something Slippery and Sticky stood out!!!*** I decided it was the very same thing as what is called Yin Essence in the Eastern Medicine. I was literally flabbergasted, for it suggested to me that the mysterious healing power hidden in those exotic plants was indeed the Yin to balance out the excesses of the Yang and render the body free from disease, just as the Traditional Chinese Medicine and/or the Traditional Eastern Medicine teaches, as I have been a student and later a practitioner of the Eastern Medicine a number of years familiarized with the same ***slippery and sticky stuff,*** it made the perfect sense to me. I accept this immediately without hesitation or any doubt.

My next step was searching the ordinary food items richly endowed with *slippery and sticky stuff* widely available in popular food markets. A cursory list of some of my favorite items will appear soon here and through Chapter 1, and again a little more detailed information is listed in Chapter 8. I wanted to provide a definite proof of my contention and theory of natural protection from diseases. I went through a series of determined daily food trials over the last several years, having started March 2012, now I have proved, to my own personal satisfaction, and in my own personal body, and report that the powerful natural healing principle hidden freed me, literally cell by cell, tissue by tissue, from my sinus congestion and the related morbidities that tortured me over five decades. How do I know? I know because I experienced personally in my own body from day to day, month to month, and year to year. The digestive tract took the longest: six full years, and ongoing. I was wondering what was going on. Then one day something that I dubbed later as "a memorable event" occurred. (This was a euphemism of a life-long blockage at the distal end of the digestive tract finally having been cleared.) I felt this event finally relieved me of a lifelong obstruction of chronic dehydration. You see the lack of proper hydration caused my body to continue to stay dehydrated no matter how often or how much water I had diligently drunk.

I have finally proved my hypothesis that something "slippery and sticky" in my nutrition was essential for proper hydration to occur. And I also learned that the Proper Hydration is the Mother Nature's Secret Key of ensuring the humanity of lifetime health and freedom from disease. I belatedly realized this after much suffering, and I also realized belatedly that the many human races around the globe are probably losing touch with once their closely guarded ancestral traditional diet in similar way as happened in relentless continuous push for modernization to the small riverside village in which I grew up in South Korea. The once fertile vegetable gardens and fruit orchards of my father's time on fertile alluvial soil, which was appropriately called Keun Deul, or Great Field, has now been completely erased and turned into sets of dense suburban city blocks!!!

I eventually learned that this "something slippery and sticky" was the crucially essential stuff that successfully removed my 50 years long chronic disease handily and restored my full health remarkably, as I was approaching this old body's 80th birthday. I learned true and proper hydration of my body, or your body, or anybody else's, does not occur just by drinking water, as we are told.

I figured out that ... (Pardon me for using bold print for emphasis.)

...the earliest human ancestors' diet was apparently full of grass and or any green plant stuff, so that their esophagus must have stayed fully smeared by *"slippery and sticky stuff"* practically all the time by their habitual diet. (Don't you agree?)

...so that whenever they obtained clean water from nature and drank it, it must have washed down some of the stuff on the walls of their esophagus and gets mixed in with, which formed the characteristic "body water" by the time it reached the stomach. This step allowed water from the nature to turn organic which helped apparently make our bodies to be free from inflammation, disease and pain due to disease.
...and which was over time likewise engineered by the wisdom of our ancestral living bodies, so that our digestive, heart and blood circulation, growth and reproduction, health maintenance including mental health, and with male and female sexualities, for successful as well as enjoyable copulations anytime desired and generate new offspring; so that various essential body functions adapted, adjusted and formulated in infinitesimal forms and ways various potential diseases successfully overcome many times and afford us a long living privilege, all of it points singularly to this smear with *"slippery and sticky stuff"* on the walls of the esophagus. Ultimately, it is Mother Nature's free water turned organic, allowed properly nourish the living human body.

So if you are truly devoted to our ancestral traditional heritage you can pursue and successfully persist in a disease free lifetime as long as you live just by making sure that you leave enough smear of that *"slippery and sticky stuff"* on the walls of your esophagus. Eat this stuff all the time-- just keep this in your mind-- all the time!!!

After that it progressed rather quickly. Within a few months any sign of sinus congestion was completely gone and the most persistent problems of hard of hearing and watery eyes finally got cleared. Sniffles persisted longer but I know it will be eventually ceased. And even my somewhat deteriorated memory, I hope, I may help myself stabilized at a level to maintain my life independent and functional as I have been so far. I cook my own meals every day and take a walk out of doors once or twice per day, 1 to 3 hours most every day.

Throughout this long and tedious process I most prominently conquered my nemesis that has tortured me nearly 50 years with no medication. I just had experienced some delayed healing described above in fine prints. I repeat "with no medication whatsoever." And the result was: No more nasal congestions, no more polyps, no more itchy eyes, no more hard of hearing in any of my ears, all of these troubles of chronic sinus congestion have completely cleared out naturally without using any hint of medication except my very simple natural food diet. So, that's my story of complete personal victory wrested over one of the most difficult diseases that controlled my life nearly 50 years.

Looking back at what I did during the last 8 years (and continuing) was a step-by-step restoration process of my body's Yin deficiency status. By using modern terminology, what I did was proper step by step rehydration of my body over the 8 years, (and continuing until the end of my life) and thus correcting and then restoring physiological damages wrought on my body over my entire earlier life by repeated "hydration failures" every time I drank water throughout my earlier lifetime without what I consider to be the necessary condition *sine qua non* for proper hydration to be successfully achieved, that is, without adequate amount of Yin, or soluble fiber in my nutrition. There is absolutely nothing more basic and important than water to human or any life for that matter, but the absolute need of water to be coupled with this necessary nutrition still is largely shrouded under confusion or no one else talk about the need in our societies. The consequences of my lifetime hydration failures resulted in unchecked dehydration of my body, a chronic disease status termed Chronic Yin Deficiency in the Eastern Medicine. It took me more than 8 years with the proper nutrient to accomplish proper hydration throughout my body and restore the damages done by hydration failures accumulated throughout my entire life. And in the process, I think I gained an intimate experience and knowledge showing some light into **how successfully the evolving humanity should have negotiated with Mother Nature for a disease-free sustainable life on earth for the entire humanity.** This conclusion of mine is completely replicable to any person interested in simply by repeating my protocols or eating the foods I suggest. Although I spent more than 6 to 8 years of time to prove the same, one can experience some important benefits much sooner, if one tried. If you had a sleeping disorder or erectile failure, for example, either problem may be quickly resolved within a month or two, or permanently as long as continuously using the suggested food. These may appear like miracles to some. No more myths on the subject of sleeping disorder or erectile failure shall be sustainable once this book is out and read by everyday people, for the result of taking this nutrition shall be so quick, stark, and so satisfyingly fulfilling. I hope you will begin to realize that we are indeed the beings raised ultimately by Mother Nature. Our life and death, from the very beginning of this world, to the very end of it, if there is one going to be, will be the Mother Nature.

Here I am so sure of myself that I feel I must challenge every reader to replicate my own experience in your very own personal satisfaction and prove it to yourself that the mucilage rich foods indeed protect you from disease and pain – potentially any and all diseases, except those caused by using non-food items, or drugs such as opioids. We may have reached an Armageddon of drugs. The only viable exit strategy from this will be a complete return eventually back to the Mother Nature's PROTECTION. If you suffer from disease or pain, please try to replicate my successful experiment – toward your own lasting health and happiness.

I want to return now back to my focus on the broad subject of a disease-free sustainable life on earth for the entire humanity. I know now this plain natural and existential fact of humanity is shrouded in the dark by dead silence of the scientific community. **As a result, the masses do not understand that they can stay free from disease by Mother Nature, or simply by eating foods that contain proper nutrients, or by practicing the self-care of prevention. Instead, they stay in the dark and suffer from various diseases.** In our society, a scientist, professor, doctor, and lawyer have been traditionally respected as a professional operating on certain level of professional standards and on their conscience. Now as society diversifies one can hire a lawyer for any cause one may care about as long as he is willing and able to pay, and as the so called healthcare is considered one of the top money maker businesses and has become a proper and a coveted domain of an investor. An investor is in business with a goal of multiplying his money to the maximum extent it is possible. And that investor may often sit on the very top and can make and break any proposed research project in healthcare. In this kind of set up, no one seems eager to talk about the free natural protection from disease, available to everyone, rich or poor, and free of charge. So, there may be a silent stalemate. I dare hopefully to break the silence for there is the health of the humanity at stake. I say plainly *"Mother Nature's help is here and now, by way of simple nutrition, and is available to you practically free of charge!"* I hope starting a conversation that will eventually lead people to get familiarized with the Mother Nature's protection on how she takes care of us all to stay free of disease and/or pain.

Two Young Men's Plight Tugs at My Heart

"Nasal mucous membrane chronically swollen" can be very difficult to manage. I know that from my personal history over 40 years. One desperate man posted on the Internet asking, "Has anybody successfully tried medications to treat chronically swollen nasal mucous membranes?" It's the same type of condition that I have suffered from for over 40 years. Apparently, there is no effective treatment available even in England/ or the United Kingdom, technologically one of the world's most advanced countries. It may be one of the most misunderstood and demeaning health conditions for the sufferer as well. He alone suffers in the night in his bed because he can't breathe, and it makes sleeping difficult if not impossible. In the morning he can get up and go to work because he has to. He often may fall asleep at work. His boss and coworkers may think he's just lazy or neglects his duty as I had experienced at my work. Even his wife after weeks and months may get tired of him. He lost his humor if there was any. There are few options for him. (I am not writing about any specific person here, but just extrapolating out of my own past experiences.) Two such young men posted the following messages and I happened to notice them. I haven't had any contact with them. I hope they will hear about my book and it will be helpful to them and many others like them.

Accessed 7/15/2013
Science Forums
www.science-bbs.com
Author Boris Holla: Nasal mucous membranes chronically swollen
Has anybody successfully tried medications to treat chronically swollen nasal mucous membrane?
My ENT specialist diagnosed hyperplastic conchae nasalis. Allergy test was negative. I have difficulty in getting enough air especially at night. He recommended conchotomia and septum correction. I haven't undergone surgery yet because
1. I don't understand what the septum correction good for. If it is bent to one side, the hole at the opposite side should get better ventilation, thus total ventilation wouldn't improve.
2. The reason why I don't get enough air through my nose is, IMO, the swollen mucous membrane, which won't be cured by surgery. I do get enough air if I use nasal spray. Besides I do know some people who had undergone surgery and had the same problem some years later.
Nasal sprays containing alpha-agonists like xylometaziline or ephedrine work for a while but are not suitable for long term use since they cause receptor degradation and atrophy of mucous membrane.
I tried hoisting water and salted water into the nose, but this worsened it.
Inhaling improves ventilation for 1-2 hours.
Boris Hollas

Author Amit Steiner: Nasal mucous membrane chronically swollen
Hi,

I have a similar condition, and I had all possible treatments, including nasal cortico steroids, local and general antihistamines, cromolyn, alpha agonists, and a combination of all. None made any good, except systemic alpha agonists which are not a cure …

Apart from this, I have had conchotomy about a year ago. I had been convinced by my ENT specialist that it will bring ULTIMATE improvement in two weeks at most. "free breathing" he called… 12 months has [sic] passed – everything is about the same. Nothing has improved since then.

To say, I've lost belief in ENT's over the last year. They all say contradicting stuff. Most said I had a 'successful' operation', and while others said it was a failure and that I need another one …

I guess I'm one of those cases which are too big a challenge for ENT docs …

Reading these stories revives my painful memories of hopelessness I went through five decades ago. I was told I had allergic rhinitis, which blocked my nasal breathing completely. In the night in the wee hours, I had asthma attacks, which made me struggle hanging my head downward from bed in an effort to keep the airway open in my throat and fighting that suffocating strangulation torturing me with incessant coughing as well. Night after night! A true living nightmare! And in the morning I had to get up and go to work. I was a young married man with a four-year-old boy. Fortunately, we found a Head Start childcare center in uptown Chicago, which was free, thanks! My allergist had given up treating me with medication. None of her so-called allergy de-sensitizing treatments, nor the subsequent antibiotics and then boosted mega-doses of them seemed to make any difference at all. Finally, she shook her head defeated and sent me to an ENT. The ENT doc turned out to be a Korean man. Could surgery help? I asked. It might not, but if you ask me, I'll do it, he said. I probably knew at the time as a patient that an ENT's surgery was unlikely to help me because my case was based on allergy. But one of those two young men appears to have submitted to the surgery fully trusting his reassuring doctor, and that's what it hurt the most, and forty years after my debacle. Saying that I was shocked would be an understatement. I was deeply saddened. I felt strongly that those young people should have been properly helped in their health problems so that they could concentrate on bettering their own lives and that of their loved ones. For what happened to me in the 1970's happened again to these young men and potentially many others 40 years later in the 2010's according to the reports on the Science Forums quoted above.

In recollection of my case, after the surgery was done and I came to I was sent back home, and the next week when the gauze stuffing was removed from my nasal cavities, I had expected I should be able to breathe freely at last. But it was not to be. There was not a scintilla of difference before and after. Not even a single moment of comfort experienced! I was brought back exactly where I started. It was a terrible let down. I felt I should be able to do something to address this but there was none I could think of. There was just a void or emptiness. A void in your heart demands to be filled up, with an act or something. I chose to get another surgery. This time at a well respected university hospital in Korea. Would that make any difference? The difference was that I wasn't put under general anesthesia. Other than that, it was the same disappointment all over again. I regretted it was foolish of me. All these painful memories have rushed back to me as I write this.

Chapter 1

YING YANG COMES TO THE FOREFRONT

What am I talking about with 3,000 years old concept and verbiage like Yin-Yang stuff? In my opinion, Yin-Yang is not outdated but very current. Besides it has the advantage of simplification, and the 3,000 plus years old unchanged and constant meaning, as I'll soon explain it. I believe, that the basics of the Yin-Yang theory that says the warming effect of Yang and the cooling effect of Yin needed to be in balance so that health may result in the body, is still true today, and that is constant and unchanged. Although today's nutritional and medical sciences are far advanced from the time of Eastern Medicine came into being, the basic idea of balance between the two contrasting opposite forces at work seems to be sound to me and still applicable. Therefore, I made it my task to identify what was supposed to be the Water, or Yin Food, and what was to be the Fire, or Yang Food. As matter of fact, although we have had contrasting classifications of Yin herbs and Yang herbs for hundreds or thousands of years, the Eastern Medicine has never addressed or inquired the kind of specific questions that I am asking about our today's foods. I might say this was simply not its mode of inquiry, or it may be simply that no one came to ask this kind of question, as medicine tended to be professionalized as it progressed, and any food questions were let naturally fall into the household women's domain. But when I decided that I would "make my food as my medicine and make my medicine as my food," I felt I had to be able to pinpoint which specific food should represent the ultimate Yin or the ultimate Yang character, so that by balancing those two characters of foods I should be able to attain health automatically just by eating them in a balanced proportion as the ancient scientific theorist may have envisioned. As I set out in earnest to find them, seriously, for I often tended to imagine the man may also have been an ancient caveman stargazer as well, a sort of a well-rounded man of science as well as practical life experiences.

Fortunately, for me there were hints and clues in our current nutritional sciences that would readily link to my Yin Yang Metabolic Reactor. Thus, the all those three so called major nutrients, carbohydrates, fats, and proteins are ultimately broken down into glucose to be absorbed into the body.

YANG = FIRE (Calorie producing foods)   YIN = WATER (Produces cooling effect)
Carbohydrates   Mucilage
Protein   (or fiber dissolved in water)
Lipids

Diagram 1. Yin Yang Metabolic Reactor

Glucose is the fuel for the body, and produces energy when combined with oxygen, which is a chemical way of describing of making fire. The amount of energy thus produced is counted in terms of calories, or units of heat. Therefore, I'll accept all these three calorie producing foods as largely equivalent to what I call Yang/ Fire Food. And as for its opposite contrarian would be non-calorie producing food, I accept Yin=Water and read it as practically identical to mucilage water or fiber dissolved in water. And I see this to be the common essence of all Yin tonic herbs of the Eastern Medicine such as tienmendong (asparagus tuber), maimendong (ophiopogon tuber), shashen (radix glehniae), etc. etc. If you soak one of these Yin rich herbs in water, you will see its mucilage leaching out, slippery to touch at first, and then after a while moisture evaporates it will get sticky on your fingers. This is the Yin Essence as traditionally known because all Yin herbs share these slippery and sticky characteristics. In fact, all living plants share these characteristics to some degree because all plants contain some mucilage more or less. Mucilage is soluble fiber dissolved in water. I will call it from now on either mucilage or soluble fiber. Mucilage or soluble fiber is the opposite contrarian to calorie producing foods. For example, enough of regular consumption of mucilage or soluble fiber is likely to protect the body against diabetes by slowing down digestion of glucose. Such an energetic balance between the two opposite contrarians is required for good health to be maintained. It is, therefore, my supreme goal to maintain this energetic balance of the calorie producing Yang Food against non-calorie producing Yin Food as explained here.

This is my logic for eating enough of what body uses but not much more than that in the long run. A good appetite is an important precondition of health. But an untamed appetite can work to ruin the health and make life miserable for a long time, or even the rest of one's lifetime. Sometimes we may get tempted. We all know this. This is a really tricky and serious danger. We should always let our conscious mind present and make an appropriate decision. A simplified formula like this will be helpful for us to stay on balance and in good health. A lifetime good health is not a pipe dream but something within our means as long as we let our conscious mind steer the course.

That's it! Really simple and easy!
Let's our conscious mind steer the course: Always!
-- Today, tomorrow, and every day!

What drove me in this quest was my understanding and appreciation that the human body has developed a very well adapted, highly sophisticated and extremely durable system that could withstand varied challenges and considerable stresses, acquired self-healing capabilities, and had a potential to live almost indefinitely and stay healthy, if lived true to its evolutionary primordial features of foods, because without such capabilities man could have long perished as dinosaurs did. This is not to ignore individual differences such as allergies, certain developmental differences and myriad of environmental factors that threaten our lives. In spite of all that we humans proved to be the most durable and successful animal on earth and arguably the ruler of all earthlings, although I have qualms about the implications of my last phrase.

And it was another concomitant assumption that the main reason why we see a proliferation of all kinds of serious degenerative diseases in relatively recent years in the so called developed industrialized societies around the globe was that our diet is at variance from the important features of our primordial foodstuffs. And I was greatly motivated to find out what those features were specifically, for I believed that if we lived true to those primordial features of food, we would be able to steer clear of most if not all of those modern diseases.

In helping me to proceed in this line of thinking, was the inspiration from Eastern Medicine, also known as the Traditional Chinese Medicine, or the Traditional Oriental Medicine, which says in a well-worn phrase, "Food and medicine (are) of the same source." And I also took inspiration from the famous phrase attributed to Hippocrates as I quoted earlier. There were also a number of other sources of inspiration, too, of recent times. When I read news articles on health, I found many of them talk about beneficial effects of fiber in the diet, helping slow down digestion and thus lowering sugar concentration in the blood stream, which helps diabetic patients avoid as many peaks of sugar load they used to suffer from, and which could help them freed eventually from that degenerative disease. Other articles also reported that fiber in the diet helps lowering inflammation in the blood vessels, thus reducing plaque formation and atherosclerosis, and thus reducing incidence of heart disease. They also reported that those who took fiber in their diet had the reduced chances of getting cancer. In reading these stories I get the impression that these reports are now accepted virtually as factual among the many medical researchers.

I repeatedly read those articles again and again. None of them were original articles but when I read them, they all said in a nutshell, "Fiber slows down digestion, and reduces inflammation," or something like that. I formulated that simplified sentence and noticed a striking similarity to what the Eastern Medicine says about Yin. Being cool in its nature, "Yin slows down digestion, and cools off Heat." The term Heat in Eastern Medicine is clinically identical to inflammation/infection as I mentioned earlier. Let me put the two sentences one after another to dramatize the similarity between them:

Yin slows down digestion and Cools off Heat. *From ancient Eastern Medicine*
Fiber slows down digestion and reduces inflammation. *From modern Western Medicine*

The juxtaposition of the two sentences from two entirely different disciplines as given above, which originated each in a time span of 2,000 years apart or even farther, is very interesting to say the least. It shows what the two distinct traditions say are remarkably similar or identical at least in this respect. Now you see that the phrase "Cools off Heat" in Eastern Medicine actually means "reduces inflammation." When both statements are true, and they are, I can safely say, by the power of syllogism, "Fiber equals Yin, and Yin equals fiber."

Fiber = Yin = Fiber (dissolved in water), also known as mucilage

Now you get the idea, that Yin-Yang is known since ancient times, that when they act, they antagonize against each other, and end up in a balanced state as long as things go well as intended.

But is that really so? Logically, I felt fiber was most likely it. This was a moment of great breakthrough for me, at least potentially. But I couldn't explain it, for I thought Yin was Water, literally, and as far as I knew at the time fiber was solid matter. Therefore, I met a stumbling block, and it sat there unmoved for some time. Then one day I punched "dietary fiber" on my laptop and hit Enter. Then I learned that mucilage was a kind of water or liquid in which soluble dietary fiber was dissolved in suspension, and this kind of fiber can absorb and hold a thousand times of water by weight. Bingo! This was it! This was what I had been looking for all along. I was sure of it!

What I have done here is I simply connected the dots, for every element in this my argument was well known and widely accepted as truth, one in the East and the other in the West. In other words, the East and the West have met here, and they both agreed as I have reported, and I will repeat it right here:

Yin slows down and Cools off Heat. *From ancient Eastern Medicine.*
Fiber slows down digestion and reduces inflammation. *From modern Western Medicine.*

(Read frequently by me piecemeal)

The Eastern and ancient tradition mostly sees it as Water, while the Western and modern tradition looks right through the water at the microscopic plant tissue components made of some protein and polysaccharides, or glycoprotein, and calls it fiber. Cut through any living plant or fruit and you get to see immediately it bleed, not in red blood, but in plant body liquid, "jinye" in Chinese, you may call it juice, or water, and that's what we call mucilage. I might choose to call it the 'essence of green plants' because it occurs in all green plants. It is plant blood equivalent because all plant nutrients are dissolved in the mucilage or 'liquid essence', and delivered, through its vascular system, to different parts of the plant body. Every plant on earth and some soil bacteria produce and depend on some. All good soil contains plenty of it. In fact, without plenty of mucilage in the dirt, plants won't do very well because mucilage helps plants retain water in their bodies, and helps roots suck in more water into the plant tissues, and plant seeds with mucilage in their seed shells when in touch with damp soil in the night will attract water and swell, and hold on it so that it can sprout in time

At the very bottom of a plant life, the lynchpin factor is its ability to attract, absorb, hold, and deliver water to different parts of the plant body. I think the mucilage in the plant tissues plays that role by interfacing the plant body vis-à-vis free water available in the nature where the plant's roots can reach. Call it evolutionary biotechnology or secrets of life. Either way, evolutionarily speaking, it seems likely that plant made use of freely available material in the soil produced by soil bacteria, that is, mucilage.

Stretch the imagination another giant evolutionary step, and, millions of years later, when animals started to appear on earth what would they eat? Well, they ate plants and plants gave them mucilage. And the mucilage finds a role to play in the body of an animal because the animal needed something to help it retain water, a large amount of it, for various functions in its body, let alone for its own body's growth. Some animals grew humongous bodies. Much of those bodies' weight consisted of water. To help them manage bodies with large amount of water the mucilage was handy to let them do so, apparently. Thus, the role of mucilage has become integral in the human body. We may have been oblivious of the fact. As long as the humanity faithfully depended on their traditional food no problem has occurred. But with so called Industrial Revolution a polishing machine was introduced most likely the very first time since human evolution in the year of 1890 A.D. The devastating tragedy that unfolded is now a well forgotten long history. **But the fact of the nutritional requirement remains unchanged for the humanity.** As a result, we are challenged to educate every individual of every new generation. With the prestige of the traditional diet eroded as it is today the task of educating our youngsters to include more fiber in their food has become a nearly impossible task to accomplish. The youngsters may have overcome the B-vitamin deficiencies by taking supplements, but that history and their dietary habit probably left them in their later life subject to diseases caused by dehydration, in my opinion, such as insomnia and erectile failure, and potentially some of the increased gynecological health troubles of modern day young women such as premature menopausal symptoms and/or vaginal dryness. (My mother used to grumble of having to deal with her menstruation in her 60's, putting out her rags on the clothe line to dry, while some younger women of her junior by two decades were struggling with their pre-menopausal syndromes.) Here, the point I want to emphasize, is the diet, the difference of my mother's lifelong dietary habit and that of modern junior women. I mean, *the diet is the sole determining factor here.* I mean I say, change your dietary habit, and shall be changed your menstrual pattern. It is as simple as that. **By the same token, if you are a young woman (a teenage girl included) plagued with gynecological troubles you should probably examine your dietary habit with emphasis on mucilage/ dietary fiber I talk about throughout this book. The mucilage/ dietary fiber was the most prominent feature of our human ancestors, has become permanently incorporated in human physiology, and has become the core human health self-protection system, or, The Mother Nature's Permanent Natural Human Health Protection. This natural protection is as durable as your personal adherence to your own habitual dietary regimen on your daily mucilage/ dietary fiber consumption. If you want this protection, you must make that choice every mealtime.**

That's the cost. The potential benefits, you figure out.

Chapter 2

WATER IS AN ESSENTIAL NUTRIENT

Human ancestors were not an exception about the water need. Water was indispensable as well as essential in every facet of a living body, including breathing, digestion, nutrient absorption, distribution, growth, reproduction, excretion, or whatever you name it. But before I can get into it I must first address a question: "Is water one of the major macronutrients for human body?" for I have never seen in my experience water being listed as a nutrient, let alone a macronutrient but my Yin-Yang model calls for water to be identical to Yin. I typed the question and searched the Internet and I got this very precisely worded and comprehensive article as an answer:

Water as an essential nutrient: the physiological basis of hydration
E Jequier (1) and F Constant(2)
European Journal of Clinical Nutrition (2010) **64,** 115-123; doi: 10. 1038/ejcn; published online 2 Sept. 2009
Abstract
How much water we really need depends on water functions and the mechanisms of daily water balance regulation. The aim of this review is to describe the physiology of water balance and consequently to highlight the new recommendations with regard to water requirements. Water has numerous roles in the human body. It acts as a building material; as a solvent, reaction medium and reactant; as carrier of nutrients and waste products; in thermoregulation; and as a lubricant and shock absorber. The regulation of water balance is very precise, as a loss of 1% of body water is compensated within 24 h. Both water intake and water losses are controlled to reach water balance. Minute changes in plasma osmolarity are the main

factors that trigger these homeostatic mechanisms. Healthy adults regulate water balance with precision, but young infants and elderly people are at greater risk of dehydration. Dehydration can affect consciousness and can induce speech incoherence, extremity weakness, hypotonia of ocular globes, orthostatic hypotension and tachycardia. Human water requirements are not based on minimal intake because it might lead to a water deficit due to numerous factors that modify water needs (climate, physical activity, diet and so on.) Water needs are based on experimentally derived intake levels that are expected to meet the nutritional adequacy of a healthy population. The regulation of water balance is essential for maintenance of health and life. On an average, a sedentary adult should drink 1.5 l of water per day, as water is the only liquid nutrient that is really essential for body hydration.

Introduction

Water is the major constituent of the human body. The latter cannot produce enough water by metabolism or obtain enough water by food ingestion to fulfill its needs. As a consequence, we need to pay attention to what we drink throughout the day to ensure that we meet our daily water needs, as not doing so may have negative health effects.

Water is the main constituent of cells, tissues and organs and is vital for life (Lang and Waldegger, 1997). Despite its well-established importance, water is often forgotten in dietary recommendations, and the importance of adequate hydration is not mentioned. As a consequence, health professionals and nutritionists are sometimes confused and question the necessity of drinking water regularly: how much we should drink, how to know whether patients are well hydrated or not. (Emphasis is mine.)

I thought this article provides a timely, firm and reliable foundation in the understanding of water as a macronutrient and demonstrates everyone's need to drink enough water daily to protect their good health, for I'm convinced that many current public health issues may have something to do with dehydration including my own life's long tormentor: sinus congestion and related issues. I want to continue quoting the article to describe the roles of water in the body below.

Water as a vital nutrient: a multifunctional constituent of the human body

Water as a building material

Water, present in each cell of our body and in the various tissues and compartments, acts first as a building material. This primary function leads to nutritional recommendations, as water needs are higher during the growth period of the body.

Water as a solvent, a reaction medium and a reaction product

Water has unique properties: it is an excellent solvent for ionic compounds and for solutes such as glucose and amino acids (Haussinger, 1996). (*Omit.*) Water as a macronutrient is involved in all hydrolytic reactions, for instance, in the hydrolysis of other macronutrients (proteins, carbohydrates, lipids and so on).

Water is also produced by the oxidative metabolism of hydrogen containing substrates in the body. Theoretically, for 1g of glucose, palmitic acid and protein (albumin), 0.6, 1.12 and 0.37 ml water is produced, or for 100 kcal of energy, 15, 13, and 9 ml water is produced.

Water as a carrier

Water is essential for cellular homeostasis because it transports nutrients to cells and removes wastes from cells (Haussinger, 1996). It is the medium in which all transport systems function, allowing exchanges between cells, interstitial fluid and capillaries (Grandjean and Campbell, 2004). Water maintains the vascular volume and allows blood circulation, which is essential for the function of all organs and tissues of the body (Ritz and Berrut, 2005). Thus, the vascular and respiratory systems, the digestive tract, the reproductive system, the kidney and liver, the brain and the peripheral nervous system, all depend on adequate hydration to function effectively (Haussinger, 1996). Severe dehydration therefore affects the function of many systems and is a life-threatening condition (Szinnai *et al., 2005*).

Water and thermoregulation

Water has a large heat capacity, which contributes to limiting changes in body temperature in a warm or cold environment. Water has a large capacity for vaporization of heat, which allows a loss of heat even when ambient temperature is higher than body temperature (Motain *et al.,* 1999). When sweating is elicited, evaporation of water from the skin surface is a very efficient way to lose heat.

Water as a lubricant and shock absorber

Water, in combination with viscous molecules, forms lubricating fluids for joints; for saliva, gastric and intestinal mucus secretion in the digestive tract; for mucus secretion in the airways in the respiratory system; and for mucus secretion in the genitourinary tract.

By maintaining the cellular shape, water also acts as a shock absorber during walking or running. This function is important for the brain and the spinal cord, and is particularly important for the fetus, who is protected by a water cushion.

Thus, the article quoted above in full makes it abundantly clear how important water is in our body and I greatly appreciate the authors of this article.

But I must add a little note to the benefit of my general readers that the term "viscous molecules" looks similar to/or identical with what I describe as "mucilage" or "fiber dissolved in water", which, in my opinion, makes the proper and effective hydration possible, and thus I name it as the water's **consort** *sine qua non* inside the human body.

I advocate strongly and without equivocation that in proper hydration there must be enough of the mucilage smudge present on the walls of the esophagus so that when you drink water, it shall necessarily and without fail, wash down the enough of mucilage smudge remaining on the walls of esophagus is needed to be washed down into the stomach, and only that water mixed with enough of mucilage smudge turns into the proper body water. And this body water is the only true and proper body water, and as such this body water properly nourishes living human body tissues and cells. Thus, this kind of body water does not cause inflammation or disease in the body, but rather removes and clears any inflammation or any disease in the way if found. And I also describe the same as "slippery and sticky stuff." And I want to repeat here that only when enough of this stuff smearing your esophagus exists, so that whenever you drink water shall wash some of the smear down and gets mixed in with it, only then the water you just drank should result in proper hydration. This means good and positive to your health maintenance. Otherwise, or without enough of that smear on the esophagus, regardless however much water/ or however often you may have drunk water, the water fails to properly hydrate your body. That means it causes dehydration in your body such as constipation, and if you have any other chronic disease it will cause to deepen it. In my opinion, proper hydration is not just about drinking water and its full implications are thus far reaching toward our lifetime health and self-health maintenance. And if you make a proper habit to accomplish proper hydration possible every time you drink water it should work to improve your health little by little over the years, chipping away your any existing organic diseases. The descriptions on this long paragraph represent the complex processes of my mental reasoning precisely, and I confess that I do not make use of any physical tools for my reasoning.

I Found the Missing Link in My Diet

In recent years I have gradually become convinced that the established medicine apparently missed something that is critical in my life and determined to find the missing link in my foods. I am confident now that I have finally identified the missing link in my nutrition. This is the most widely distributed form of nutrients and practically covers the whole earth, or in other words, ubiquitous, the land area where plants and bacteria grow as well as all surface waters where planktons and algae grow, and as such is not usually recognized as an essential nutrient but just plainly ignored. But I believe that the ancient teachers of the Eastern Medicine happened to recognize this and called it Yin. And this nutrient is found in every living plant at different levels, while in some it is found extremely rich and in others may not be so much, or I can say truly universal but distributed in varying degrees.

Think about cutting into a juicy tomato or a cucumber, for example. You see its juice flow immediately. Smear some on your fingers. It rubs slippery between your fingers, but a few moments later when the moisture decreases it gets sticky. This is the classic character: slippery and sticky in ordinary people's terms, or viscous and elastic as described by some academics. This is the typical way as mucilage is often described, and defined according to my dictionary, (Merriam Webster Collegiate Dictionary Tenth Edition) as a gelatinous substance of various plants that contains protein and polysaccharies and is similar to plant gums. Would you believe me if I told you this everyday substance turned out to be the very type of the food that represented the missing link toward my health? Yes, that is literally true, but with just one catch: It's more than that. It's a great deal more than that, because this mucilage looks like something that got involved with living things at the very beginning of life on earth, and ever since, continued through evolution, and human life was set just a little part of the whole process. The process, therefore, tied human body to the mucilage for proper hydration as it did with other animals and plants. In recent years some lip service was paid to it as water soluble fiber but in my opinion, it is far inadequate. Consequently, there is public confusion about the correct concept of effective hydration.

Now Is the Time to Make
<u>The Issue of Hydration</u>
Crystal Clear and Not Obscured

It is true to say water hydrates human body. But if you say that's all there is to it, you are wrong. Although doctors simply tell us to drink more water there is still dehydration going on even if you may drink water diligently, or even *aggressively*. I read about some senior citizens suffer from dry mouth syndrome and are unable to produce saliva in their mouths and as a result can't chew or even swallow foods. This should be a proof positive that simply drinking water alone is unable to accomplish true and effective hydration in your

body. But this phenomenon is explained away (really?) that this is a kind of mysterious incurable chronic dehydration syndrome. **To me this apparent clinical impasse should serve as proof positive that water alone is unable to properly and effectively hydrate human body. You are probably unaware that there is an obscure** *sine qua non* **condition to effective hydration, which few people seem to be familiar with these days. Unless and until this condition is fully met no effective hydration can occur to the human body. No exceptions! But be patient and read on!**

For your information, the obscure substance is one of the most widely distributed in nature and known as mucilage. As such mucilage has always been a part of a living body ever since the beginning of life on earth, first created by a soil bacterium, readily adopted by all plants and then by all plant eating animals, and therefore rightly is considered organic matter. But water is different. Water found in nature we prefer pure and free from any contamination. Therefore, the drinking water taken from nature that contains no organic matter dissolved in it should be identified as inorganic.

And what happens if you just drank a cup of such water? *It depends on your nutritional habit.* I can suggest the result may be either of the two hypothetical extremes or somewhere in between depending on food residues found on the walls of your esophagus that were washed down by the water. *Did you know this? The water taken from nature and drunk into your body sits exactly between the two very distinct worlds---- organic or inorganic.* If it found enough of organic matter chiefly of mucilage or soluble fiber dissolved in it, then the water has turned into organic when it reaches your stomach by washing down the mucilage found on the walls of your esophagus and that would be the normally expected outcome under traditional dietary habit. *And this is good because only the organic water alone can fully hydrate the body properly and protect it from disease.* What if it found little mucilage when it washed down the esophagus? In that case the water should remain inorganic just as it was introduced, and therefore the inorganic water is unable to properly hydrate an organic body. As a result, your body is unable to receive the benefit of hydration. The end result is dehydration of your body in progress, which effectively terminates the balanced state of Yin and Yang of your body, and initiates a diseased state of your body, rendering your body susceptible to inflammation. Please understand that as long as you maintain Yin and Yang at a balanced state your body is practically free from disease. I believe we can maintain this balanced state of Yin and Yang, that is free from disease, yes, I mean it, indefinitely as long as you are faithful on your diet, and its first necessary step is the realization of full hydration. **But a full proper hydration is possible only if the precondition *sine qua non* is fully satisfied, that is, your esophagus is flush with the organic matter such as mucilage or soluble fiber dissolved in it from your regular dietary habit. Lifetime health and strength may sound to you now as something enormously challenging. But I say that there is an easy and simple way via Mother Nature's grace. Satisfy the nature's simple requirement for proper hydration. Just maintain a dietary habit described above so that anytime you drink water there remains a plenty of slippery and sticky stuff on the walls of your esophagus so that whenever you drink water it can get mixed in with while it is going down. This process makes a huge difference because it renders the water from nature which is inorganic into organic. I believe that only this organic water is able to truly hydrate the body, and the inorganic water introduced and remains inorganic is unable to hydrate the body, and instead causes dehydration and over time may cause chronic dehydration. And all chronic diseases may be ultimately caused by or linked to dehydration or by failure of proper hydration. Therefore, I declare any confusion over proper hydration intolerable for the people's health and by ensuring proper hydration one can stay free from diseases indefinitely. This old truth has been under long-long obscurity hidden by the tribal customs and dietary habits.**

I assume that in the traditional diet with its enough of mucilage, water was routinely accepted by the body and processed normally, but with some modern diet from which most source of mucilage were removed such as white bread or white rice, and with little vegetables and fruits eaten as is the custom of modern young people, water cannot find enough mucilage to be mixed in with while going down the esophagus, an abnormal state starts taking place, for the water introduced is found unfit to serve the organic body. Let's assume that with subsequent meals the nutrition habit remained unchanged indefinitely. Let's just further assume the subject continued drinking a number of cups of water daily believing the practice will help hydration. If you believed you could hydrate your body this way, I want to say to you: **"It's not the way nature works. Nature requires that your esophagus is full of mucilage to be mixed with the water whenever you may drink during the day. I believe strongly this was the way ever since the beginning of any animal life on earth due to the environmental conditions that the green plants were largely their food and they were full of mucilage in them."** I strongly believe, as scientists tell us, that our earliest human ancestors preferred to live near shallow shoreline and subsisted with simple basic diet of whatever they might have been able to scrape off the land or catch in its close environs including lots of green plants, fruits, seeds, small land animals, various water plants, fish and shellfish. Although the most reliable source of their basic food, rain or shine, year after year and all year around might have been largely plants and water, and thus incorporating the mucilage, the plant essence, as the essential tool for self-preservation protection. I believe this was a miraculous biotechnology, and one of many secrets of life that allow us disease free from generation after generation.

In a modern developed society of the new generations as the traditional large family structure in which grownups and married siblings lived together with their aging parents fell out of favor, and more and more newly married siblings preferred to live separately in their own households near their jobs, the traditional foodstuffs were often shunned either due to their complexity of preparation or the lack of familiarity and eventually got lost completely. Thus, the young families find their foodstuffs where they live and work and probably nobody told them about how important it was to get some of the organic matter such as mucilage or soluble fiber. If nobody told you about this before, I want you to keep this in mind for this is the most critical piece of information for proper hydration and therefore for natural health keeping for life. Think about that. To live healthy naturally is not difficult, but to do so without proper hydration is IMPOSSIBLE! For this information is not widely shared at this time, to say the least, you can consider it as a secret just shared with you.

Self-Nurturance, or Self-Care, is the Way to Go!

We humans have survived on earth literally over countless generations. On the one side of this fantastic success story, I see the genetic strength of our human stock and the adaptability of our inherited bodies, and on the other side our ancestral tradition of sticking to the tried-and-true dietary requirements passed down generation after generation. Hidden from our view behind all of these has been the permanent protection by Mother Nature secure, which is accomplished only when proper hydration occurs. In my understanding, proper hydration is probably the path where an anti-inflammatory action takes place, which helps keep our bodies free from getting diseased. And I have to wonder who was the man that said Yin=Water 3,000 years ago. I tend to picture him as a caveman star gazer and a wise man. I try in this book to popularize an alternative path of obtaining the necessary mucilage rich foods so that no one may be left behind out of the dietary necessity, and thereby out of the Mother Nature's protection. If you choose to live by self-nurturance, I will explain how the natural protection by Mother Nature may likely pan out to protect your health all the way throughout your life in the following chapters.

Perhaps One of the Greatest Evolutionary Miracles

First of all, food is the medicine for humanity. Our daily diet needs to be recognized as our daily small miracles that have kept us *"alive and kicking,"* if not entirely trouble free, through the ages. The miracle continues every time we eat and sleep. Think about it so that we should appreciate it and do so with a clear goal of lifetime disease-free self-maintenance in mind.

Our daily miraculous meals should be the foundations on which we stand for our healthy body and healthy mind. When the food goes down the mysterious tube it's turned around through a process called metabolism into our blood, flesh, and more fresh energy for another day. Recent studies show: (1) Troublesome autoimmune diseases as well as; (2) Altzheimer's disease may be prevented by the gut bacteria.

(Note 1) Carolyn Gregoire: The Secret to Treating Autoimmune Disease May Lie in the Gut; Targeting Gut Bacteria May Be the Key to Preventing Alzheimer's; 02/21/17 *Healthy Living/ The Huffington Post*

(Note 2) Carolyn Gregoire: Targeting Gut Bacteria May Be The Key To Preventing Alzheimer's; 02/21/17 *Ibid.*

The great tube, the mysterious tube, or the digestive tract, may hold more secrets and we must work harder to dig more of them out. I have another ongoing food study on my own trying to get around using the ENT's recommended medication called Nasonex, which was the only game for my kind of sinus problem, because of a devastatingly adverse side effect that I felt as if my mind slipping away. Aged at mid-seventies, I immediately perceived this suspicion of mine a serious issue that demanded my immediate action. My daughter, however, strongly disagreed insisting that as she watched me and saw that I was able to follow conversations with people better since using the medication. But there was my own intimate feeling that my mind was being obliterated into darkness. I rejected my daughter's disagreement simply as uninformed, and "I must get out-a here right now!" I decided. I quit the medication after using it perhaps a little more than a year. My decision was easy and straight-forward since I knew instinctively that any chance of losing my mind and ***"getting lost into dementia" would be worse than dying outright.*** Therefore, I made it the supreme goal of my health to maintain my conscious mind to the very last moment of my life. To me, protecting my mind is the most supreme task of protecting my health as long as I live. I do not know that I would ultimately be successful in that effort for I have already some clear signs of some short-term memory loss.

Let Me Clarify a Quick Point Here Before Moving On!!!

The mixed drink of 1/3 cup of Lakewood Organic Pomegranate juice, 1/3 cup of Blue Diamond Almond Breeze Almond milk Unsweetened Original, and 1/3 cup of plain water, that totaled to one full cup, I used to address my sinus related symptoms since quitting the medication called Nasonex: I am doing very well for over a full year without any symptoms of congestion or blockage I used to have experienced in my nose, throat, ears and eyes. I consider this project very successful and feel I am extremely lucky but there was one problem I mistakenly overlooked, which was my hearing still blocked to some degree. My hearing eventually got cleared soon in the wake of "a memorable event" when the final blockage at the distal end of my digestive tract gave way, which marked the final completion of rehydration, in my opinion, over the previous life-long chronic dehydration wrought by the history of hydration failures although unwittingly so on my part. By the way, I still appreciate the almond drink and pomegranate juice for hydration. Later eventually I simplified this drink into 1/2 cup of water, 2 heaping spoonfuls of organic almond meal, and one full cup of organic pomegranate juice stirred up well with some fruit like slices of softened persimmon or kiwi fruit as my favorite drink 2-3 times per day. This made my magic drink for a long time. I must add that this was in addition to my basic dietary requirement of lifetime adequate daily consumption of mucilage or fiber dissolved in water.

MOTHER NATURE'S WATERING HOLE
FOR DISEASE-FREE TRUE HYDRATION

BASIC INGREDIENTS OF MY WATERING RECIPIES

(NOTE: I prefer certain fruits like avocado, kiwi fruit, persimmon, apricot, white nectarine and eat them mostly when they are generally well ripe to be tender on finger pressure. I also love red raspberries, mulberries and blueberries, and or goji-berries, a Chinese herb. I believe they are richly endowed in what I call "Slippery and Sticky Stuff" to Assist Proper Hydration.")

Step 1, Pick any desired fruits and any desired number of slices. Place them all in a salad bowl.

Step 2, Sprinkle one tablespoonful of either organic almond meal or flaxseed meal over the slices of fruits.

Step 3, Take one half cup of plain drinking water, and pour it over almond or flaxseed meal.

Step 4\. Take one full cup of Lakewood Pure Pomegranate Juice.

And that's it! I do not want any kind of dressing. And that's all. I love it!!!

I use this all the time either as for my hydration, or as a base of a quickie meal by just adding a few or several more ingredients.

Now going back to my discussion of the miraculous nature of our traditional diet, throughout the human earthly journey, even though there were tremendous sufferings and deaths at times, that doesn't erase the fact of the humanity's unchallenged survival through the eon to this day, arguably due to the dietary traditions carefully passed onto the next generations. This we have to accept as a hard fact, I am convinced. We must therefore give a special reverence for the tried-and-true traditional food, and not to challenge it on frivolous reasons. We should remember that we are to go on, pass the same unto our children and through another eon.

Mucilage Was There Supporting Lives in the Very Beginning of Humanity

My recommended items of food given as rich sources of mucilage or soluble fiber will help us continue to march on our humanity's nature protected diet. I have a vision for realizing practically disease-free society by way of public education based on prevention strategy for a great majority of people, perhaps 90-95 percent of people, if not all, as far as organic diseases are concerned., I mean by this the diseases caused by the ingestion of normal foods, and nothing else. This was my lesson from studying the implications of the humanity's survival over the eon. The earliest form of life on earth may have been a bacterium, 4.5 billion years ago. And another bacterium down the line somewhere created mucilage and then an explosion of lives started one after another, and that jumped into animals, by cleverly entrapping the most useful resource in nature, that is, water. Its continued progression has over the eons reached us today. It's simply mind boggling to consider the immensity of mucilage bacterium's contribution. Now it appears that the mucilage protected the trees from dehydration and helped them grow larger and larger, and the same mucilage residing in the living bodies of humans secretly protecting human bodies from all diseases unknown to most humans themselves if not all. Now we must realize the Mother Nature was protecting us all the way along via hydration of our body's molecule by molecule. How could we have not guessed that!!! It's the Mother Nature's secret now beginning to be bared.

It's the TRUTH! Well-armed with the truth, I'm not afraid. I am confident now and casting my life with mucilage at a full swing. Now that I have spent over 6-7-8 years using and studying mucilage rich foods in my personal diet, and more than a full year using my own dietary measure concurrently to replace my ENT prescribed medication called Nasonex, which I quit on my own over my concerns I explained above, I have gained full confidence that I am completely symptom free whatsoever and I feel I can go on like this indefinitely. I feel very good about it because my 79th birthday just passed 3 months ago. And that's what I am telling you now. Hereunder, I'll try to tamper down on my excitement, and try to share with you what it is all about. This is how my imagination goes:

How Mucilage Came into Being In the beginning, in the very, very beginning, there was the blazing sun and intense heat. There was frequent rain lately. It was in the primordial Earth just cooled off, and when there were hosts of bacteria growing rampantly and some very first new forms of plants were starting out. One of the bacteria created something that scientists now call mucilage. New plant life forms eagerly adopted the mucilage as their own because the plants needed water to grow and the mucilage was just the right thing to help them retain water inside the body of the plants and grow larger and larger.

How Mucilage Has Become Essential to Animals When animals came around, they needed lots of water for them to grow bigger, to reproduce, and to clean out the waste products. They could do all that thanks to the mucilage contained in the plants they ate as their food. The soluble fiber dissolved in the mucilage is so powerful that it can hold a thousand times of its own dry weight in water. That helped the animals to drink water from the nature and metabolize it so that water has become as integral part of their organic bodies, and not a foreign material. And because water and the fiber are so strongly attracted to each other that they become united as indispensable partner to each other so that water and the dissolved fiber inside the animal body behaved now almost like one single entity.

Humans Are Intelligent and Voluntary Beings Humans share all of those said above about mucilage with animals. Humans are smart and they can make their own choices unlike animals. This sometimes causes troubles for them when nature doesn't agree with them. Although their choices on diet and lifestyle are vast and wide open when something cuts directly against a physiological requirement the nature's response can be quite severe and unforgiving in cases such as this one. **In the human body, water and the soluble fiber as its consort, are united in conjugal and inseparable relationship.** That means that if the body lacks the soluble fiber the body is denied hydration, because the water drunk taken from free water in nature does not turn automatically into an organic part of the human body but should remain a foreign inorganic material unless there were enough residues of soluble fiber on the walls of the esophagus to be washed down and get mixed in with. ***Inorganic water without soluble fiber to be mixed in with remains inorganic and a foreign material, and therefore is unfit to be a part of the living body and therefore unable to hydrate it.*** Water drunk into the body turns organic only when it is mixed with enough of organic matter such as soluble fiber. This nature of water sitting between both the organic and the inorganic worlds is not well understood. In my understanding, however, there is no other way around. This should be declared a physiological fact, but it appears to me that the most Western Medicine scientists are not there at this time. This statement happens to highlight the critical importance of the traditional diet. In the traditional diet the soluble fiber was probably adequately supplied, people were blithely unaware of its need, or even less of its name, but that was O.K., because they were well taken care of. Now, however, it seems to be a different story. The times have changed. People like to try different food every day, for example. They feel rigidly pushed to offer different menu on the table at every meal and get used to operating that way from day to day, and in this kind of operation something like soluble fiber that traditionally may have come from several unremarkable or unpopular sources such as whole grains or roughage greens tend to get thinned out almost to nothing, because the whole grains and roughages are the very things that are intensely disliked and rejected outright by our new crop of young people, who are smart and increasingly self-assured. And the white flour bread and the white rice, in spite of their denuded nature of fiber, are extremely popular especially with young people to a degree that I might call it a 'fatal attraction.' Is this what is happening? I hope not but it looks it might be, I'm afraid. In large surveys increasingly younger age groups are suffering the diseases that traditionally tormented people 20-40 years older – which means an accelerated dehydration, because as people get older they tend to get further dehydrated. This is due to their dietary choices I'm explaining. The experts who apparently are not familiar with their dietary issues do not understand totally clueless and ask why.

Trend for "More Calories, Less Fiber"
Seems Set Driving Our Lives Already

I am afraid but the historical trends of moving away from the features of traditional food may have been set and appear to be no longer reversible. For example, in the year around the 1890 when grain polishing machines were invented into service, the event unleashed a devastating nutritional disaster I may call "a grain polishing syndrome" throughout the world, which continues in my opinion reverberating today worldwide. Many people in Japan and other Asian countries, who thought they were 'lucky' enough to be able to eat the most admired white rice died of vitamin B deficiency disease, or at least suffered from it. My mother, who has just passed away in January 2018 at 96, told me years ago when she had her clear memory "I had a cousin who got married to a Korean man living in Japan died because she ate the white rice, which we couldn't even afford a chance to cast our eyes on." I thought we should have learned from the debacle and properly moved on. But I realize now, with a great disappointment and shock that we merely marched in time, and what I considered a nutritional disaster settling in our lives as a new normal and permanent feature. I honestly don't know where we stand right now.

In the West where wheat is the main grain instead of rice it was white bread that was problematic. In the recent decades the problem has just begun to be addressed, or so I thought, but there seems to be still a long way to go. Consider young people in their 20's and 30's, they can't fall asleep, and ask doctors for sleeping pills. In the past, only seniors used to complain about insomnia. Do people know about this? Have today's young folks suddenly gotten older in a big jump? Many health specialists are left wondering. To me this is clear: Yin Deficiency arrived too soon by the decades definitely tied to the white flour preference food habit. They have a problem with the same dietary deficiency as I discussed above, I suspect. Consider middle aged people in their 40's and 50's, they say they have erectile failure and ask doctors for Viagra pills. These things may be mysterious to some, but it is clear to me that these are all signs of dehydration going on, signs that people's dietary habits are a-changing, or rather a new generation has dropped out of the habit of traditional food and is already losing the protective cover afforded by the traditional food. Their complaints both are caused by dehydration, or Yin deficiency in the Eastern Medicine terminology. If they don't believe what I say they should try some of the foods I talk about and see what happens. I just have to ask a rhetorical question: If the young people couldn't sleep through the nights, if the middle-aged people find their penises lay limp in the early mornings, how do you think the humanity has come to multiply and overrun the entire world as we are today? It's the Mother Nature. Our ancestors through their painstaking learning over their many lifetimes handed us the dietary traditions we have inherited. These are directly related to our health and they are indispensable treasures. Toss them away, you suffer, or even imperil your lives. They may not understand the implications of what they are doing. But they are not safe living that way. If you trust Mother Nature she would take care of you. Things like sleeping and having sex are among the essential staples for the humanity on earth. They would be almost like natural phenomena with the traditional diets. The solutions are in the diet and not in medications. If we had to depend on medications for them the days of humanity's survival on earth might be numbered. We need good stability to sustain our society and people's health serves as its core. Young forks should be taught that there are good reasons for certain features of traditional food. If they have allergy to a particular food, that would be a legitimate issue to avoid that food, but otherwise should learn to like them. They should be taught that by pushing away roughages they miss the most centrally essential health promoting nutrients although they may look like marginal foods. They are again the most important elements of our diet if you care about health and want to keep diseases at the bay.

A Massive Number of Young Folks in Dehydration

Eastern Medicine teaches that dehydration causes insomnia. Their term for dehydration is officially Yin Deficiency. I read about an interesting survey on the subject of insomnia at a website, I accessed 10/07/17, thesavvyinsomniac.com. The American Psychological Association's *2013 Stress in America* survey showed that reports of lying awake at night due to stress highest among the youngest adults and fell off as people aged. Here are the figures:

- 52% of millennials reported stress-related insomnia, as did
- 48% of gen Xers
- 37% of baby boomers, and
- 25% of seniors

Most people reading this article may say, "Wow! Half of American young people are so stressed and can't sleep!" But it comes to me at a different angle: "Wow! Half of American young people are ripe enough to be seniors!" for insomnia used to be an exclusively senior affliction, and rightly so because the typical change as people get old is getting wrinkles from dehydration, or Yin deficiency. Now what has happened? Here's what I read from it:

(1) American youth are apparently malnourished – largely due to their frivolous choice. Shocking, is it?! The major story of this article should be dehydration resulting from nutritional deficiency of soluble fiber. In my reading the cause of insomnia is dehydration and not stress. My interpretation continues in the following numbers:

(2) Due to a widely shared overwhelming sense of affluence after the wars with belt tightening off.

(3) I get the impression that in some communities this affluence is not

shared, and hunger is a daily issue, the larger society, however, is fluff with money and is soaked in a culture of wasteful ways of food handling both in commercial businesses as well as in private homes. Apparently, what is happening may be that much of the most nutritious part of fruits and vegetables peeled off and the skin was discarded; for example, carrot skin need not be peeled off, but scrubbed hard and eaten whole, and on some fruit, one need not remove a good half to 3/4 inch good to eat flesh along with the skin. Most vulnerable nutrients in discarding peels are vitamins, minerals and, especially, the fiber or the mucilage. And in the bread brown is generally disliked and white is preferred. Young Americans pre-aged enough to be counted as insomniac shows fiber deficiency because the lack of water-soluble fiber in the system will prevent proper hydration even if drinking water continued, and because insomnia will not occur if there was proper hydration in the body. Insomnia is the result of dehydration. This is how I read it. We must take these seriously as warning signals.

(4) A hopeful note: With organic gardening and farming going on strongly popular and spreading, we should counter the preceding three points and hit back at them with a movement: "Eat the whole grains with their rich store of fiber, and also eat skin and whole fruits and vegetables where you can." But I know this will likely be a hard sell because the trends of affluence are already set and going on in full steam.

Failure to Hydrate May Promote Degenerative Diseases

It is my humble opinion but, I believe that the failure to hydrate, or the on-going dehydration, even if you may keep drinking water, nonetheless, may lurk the hidden cause of proliferating so called degenerative diseases epidemic going on in this country. As an observer I find it simply scandalous that our medical community fails to grasp the basic question of effective hydration and to appreciate the urgent need of proper essential nutrients so marginalized in our society. The host of degenerative diseases proliferating in our society should be mostly prevented by promoting proper nutrition in timely manner, the very soluble fiber I am talking about, rather than wait and let the problem be festered into a huge epidemic and then let people scream "Medical treatment! Medical treatment!", as they did in recent Democratic 2020 election campaigns. Why don't we promote a dietary preventive measure, which will cost very little money and teach the people how they can help themselves?

Tackle the Huge Problem with Consumer Self Help Education

Yes! I want to encourage a consumer self-help education program so that every individual in our society shall be taught simple information to help keep themselves healthy such as consuming dietary fiber on daily basis.

I believe this kind of public self-help education program can be organized so that it shall cost little money for the community, or the individual people themselves, but is expected to reap huge health benefits society-wide that may result. We can also consider asking some non-profit donors for help educating people. I hope this effort will become a movement to change our society from desperation to prosperity by encouraging the spirit of self-help.

Globally, However,
"Something Viscous and Elastic" in Vogue!

But turn your eyes around the globe and back into the history, and you see a totally different scene there. Having studied the Eastern Medicine, starting my inquiry there was logical. As I said earlier the Yin and Yang theory is still current and helped me to clear the logjam of hydration question. Later period Eastern Medicine discussions, however, often involved long mysterious ideological arguments of the powerfully established and professionalized medicine with tenuous realistic underpinnings, typically of the so called Five Elements Theories, which often left me mystified and unconvinced. I preferred the earliest primitive beginnings of scientific inquiries into the health and disease when some thoughtful people studied the items of their diet with keen interest and acumen. We can no longer get in touch with findings by these earlier people but we can utilize some of the same and similar plant materials still used as food and or medicine in some pockets of populations. I searched for these items widely around the globe, not just in the regions of the Eastern Medicine, but possibly to get back on one of the strings of the long held dietary traditions. What resulted out of this search was apparently a common thread connecting different regions with ancient population centers widely around the globe. It's most amazing to find all these people from different regions of the globe knew what they wanted and that they agreed on one and the same kind of quality, that is, – **something viscous and elastic,** or in other words, **something sticky and slippery** – although it was sourced from various different plants. Different regions yielded different plants, and their people offered different stories like the dressed-up lore telling pharaoh's being healed by eating herb called molokheia, also known as jute, or Jew's Marrow used to make burlap, but its tender leaves have been used as specialty healing herbs, since ancient Egypt or now called Egyptian spinach in English. Both western and eastern coastal regions of Africa yielded different plants but with the same character known later to be okra and red roselle of Rwanda and brought to America by the slave traffic and popularized as Cajun diet in the southern states of Louisiana and Mississippi. Also favored by Cajuns were the broad leaves of an American tree Sassafras. Among the other lesser-known herbs in America were slippery elms of the Great Plains of Native Americans. They passed it on to early European settlers who chose to live in their neighborhood. It is amazing to me to find the same herbal character in vogue throughout Africa was sought after in America apparently long before Columbus and found 3,000 miles away across the ocean by the Native Americans in the inner bark of a tree later to be called slippery elm. Some botanical archaeologists, please join and help write out possibly the world's oldest detective story. This is the story that started when a bacterium created its first set of mucilage, which subsequently hopped on little plants, larger plants, all sizes of trees and eventually the entire vegetation both on the land as well as on the water. Some plants and trees grew hospitable to hold an exceptionally large amount of mucilage and became known as molokheia to Egyptians as well as elm tree known to the Native Americans. My story of plants favored by rich mucilage still continues.

In old Europe artichoke bulb was known as healing herb since Greece, through Rome and is still very popular today. When the Europeans crossed the Atlantic they brought the artichoke with them and have popularized it in America until today. There are several others. I'll mention just one or two more here. Flax seeds have become popular here in America in recent decades among women as menopausal symptoms reliever. Flaxseeds, also called linseeds, have a long history of being known as medicine perhaps into thousands of years, and is now being looked at as a nutraceutical or functional food. The other is also a seed, and this one very tiny. Long before I learned its name, I heard its fame with Raramuri tribal runners of Aztec people of old Mexico. They ran with one spoonful of the seeds, chewing them in the mouth, up and down the hills all day long to pass the messages of enemy attacks as the story goes. Twenty some years ago when I lived in Los Angeles around 1997-98, I was one of the volunteers serving water and banana at one of the rest stops on the foothills of Mt. Wilson, at the Angeles National Forest, for a 100 miles endurance race through the mountain trails starting from Wrightwood at 8 a.m. Saturday morning and overnight finishing at Pasadena Stadium sometime in the Sunday afternoon. Who would have guessed that I would witness at least a part of the drama that a 56-year-old Raramuri elder runner would upset and, beat a strapping young man in his mid-30's, and win the race? Watching the event, I gained more than a moral lesson, but also on health. The younger man passed our station leisurely, just a few miles to the stadium, and declined men and women offering him water and banana, knowing sure he would be the winner. A short while later though, we heard that the front runner collapsed due to dehydration, was taken to the hospital in emergency by a helicopter, and the Raramuri elder runner claimed the winner's medal. The tiny chia seeds of Aztec Indians reputedly trace back to the Mayan empire, where they were treated like gifts from gods, seemed to be the real winner to me.

Chinese Yam, Ma in Korean or scientifically Radix Dioscoreae oppositae, popularly introduced in the name of cinnamon vine to the U.S. farmers as a potato substitute in the aftermath of Irish potato failure and famine in the mid-19th century. If it were successful, today's healthcare issue in America might be perhaps far different or even non-existent. While I stayed in Korea 2010-14, I regularly bought ma from roadside vendor women, cooked and ate them. It's a specialty for a small number of health conscious following like me. The large white root looking like a baseball club is full of juice that is very slippery as well as sticky, an exemplary Yin Essence food to me and the quote below proves it. The Traditional Eastern Medicine, however, calls the dried version of the same San Yao, a Qi herb, but is silent on this valuable fresh version.

Yam is a member of the monocotyledonous family Dioscoreaceae and is a staple food in West Africa, South East Asia, and the Caribbean regions. Yam is consumed as raw yam, cooked soup, and powder or flour in food preparations. Yam tubers have various bioactive components, namely, mucin, diocin, dioscorin, allantoin, choline, polyphenols, diosgenin, and vitamins such as carotenoids and tocopherols. Mucilage of yam tuber contains soluble glycoprotein and dietary fibre. Several studies have shown hypoglycemic, antimicrobial, antioxidant activities of yam extracts. Yam may stimulate the proliferation of gastric epithelial cells and enhance digestive enzyme activities in the small intestine.

Quoted from ncbi.nlm.nih.gov, as accessed 10/20/17, Roots and Tuber Crops as Functional Foods, Int J Food Sci 2016; 2016: 3631647.

Another mucilage rich food I had in Korea was sea-green called dashima in Korean. (It's usually sold as dried sheets in stores and also known as gonpi, gombu, kunfu, or confu.) This same dried seaweed, I found in a few grocers in the U.S. and labeled as "sea tangle." I just cut them out palm sized stack of sheets and then take one per meal, chopped into smaller pieces, throw them at bottom of my cooking pot along with other items on the top. Because their usual way was to draw a light broth for seafood soup and then discard the whole thing, I thought much of the good food was wasted that way. Although some say cooking it longer draws out flavor that is not fashionable, I didn't mind that at all. I mostly cared about consuming the soluble fiber in it and enjoy it every time I eat it. I also bought through the mail flaxseeds, and chia seeds, in 5 lbs sacks, and used them interchangeably as one of the equally rich mucilage source foods mentioned above. And I bought through mail two 1 lb bags of powdered inner bark of the famous elm tree for testing at $10 each bag plus shipping. I found it dead, I mean bio-actively dead. And no mucilage released whatsoever! So, I had to throw them away. I have had a similar experience with flax and chia seeds earlier, for I had three tablespoonfuls of each, ground them in the blender with water for a drink, and was dismayed to find the resulting liquid dead! So, I learned my lesson: no more grinding, which made me prefer stone ground, in anything that is ground. But cooking in water was not a problem, and in my experience, I didn't see it damaging the mucilage. I am generally wary of buying anything ground or powdered, and prefer stone-ground, coarsely-ground, or crushed instead.

The Common Healing Properties Sought After Around the Globe

I was greatly impressed by the fact that the common healing properties were sought after around the globe from these diverse plants across the ocean and thousands of miles away, which convinced me to launch my study. What you are reading is the result of it. Enough was spilled about it so far and the answer is coming clear to most readers. The original answer, however, possibly the earliest, was already spelled out long time ago in the Eastern Medicine: Yin, a mysterious word to many of my readers. Yin is a big word as a counterpart to Yang in the Yin and Yang Theory, but here I want to use it in a limited sense on its material aspect in relevance to hydration, water and food, which are my main subjects. When I say Yin herbs, or in a step broader, Yin foods, such characterized herbs or food items are known to the Eastern Medicine as promoting hydration, thus Yin ultimately equals Water. Every new student in the Eastern Medicine dutifully memorized "Yin equals Water" without ever truly understanding its full implications, including this writer.

Here I explain the complexities involved in some dry word exercise to the new student who has never even suspected any complexities hidden underneath:

I want to revisit my dictionary at mucilage, reading: 1) "a gelatinous substance of various plants (as legumes or seaweeds) that contain protein and polysaccarieds and is similar to plant gums." 2): "an aqueous usually viscid solution (as of a gum) used especially an adhesive."

As you can see, mucilage definition 1 states a description of a chemical content analysis of mucilage exclusive of water. This kind of stuff can rarely exist in the real life except in chemist's laboratory or on his paper, because this substance is strongly attracted to water so that it can hold 1,000 times its own dry weight in water and therefore is very unstable for it to exist in nature. I call this a description of soluble fiber. Definition 2) describes it after water was added to it, or before water was removed from its original natural state. And this is the real-life mucilage: watery usually sticky and slippery like gum. See my earlier descriptions usually paraphrased the definition 2). Because I am talking about nutrition, I want to describe something people can see, touch and find it real. But my mucilage is something good to eat as food, and not something used and dedicated as adhesive.

Historically mucilage goes back all the way to the very beginning of life on earth as I explained earlier. This is soluble fiber in water solution. Several edible seed grains hold plenty of both the water soluble and insoluble fibers in their coarse seed coats. Coarsely milled or stone ground wheat, barley or oats, if they are available (I honestly don't know if they are because I am allergic to gluten and largely stay away from them. But I can use spelt safely, an ancient variety of wheat that contains some gluten. I love spelt flakes as an easy to cook whole grain.) If you are not allergic to them, they offer good amount of both fibers and therefore would-be health promoting specialty foods. One of my uncles used to say "Barley was the energy food. Without eating barley meals, you cannot do the heavy farm work," he used to say. I would encourage everyone to prefer real brown bread and real brown rice over denuded white bread or white rice to protect your health for the rest of your life. Health is your choice. Our current craze for medical treatment is vastly misdirected. Wake up, be sensible and follow the nature of your own body.

See what I said above. The substance can hold 1,000 times its own weight in water. This power controls and authorizes water to be inside the body. Did I say "auhorizes water"? Yes, I did! Not in the U.S. law, but in the body's law according to my opinion, because the earliest primordial life forms have adopted the mucilage as an essential part of their bodies and passed it on their descendants and that's how it has become an essential part of our bodies, and that is my understanding. It is going to make distinction between two different kinds of water: good body-water and illegal body-water. Good body-water has adequate soluble fiber dissolved in it. Body "hires" this substance, or married to it, and stays together as if married, to help maintain water throughout the body and maintain the body free from dehydration and free from disease. This was in the natural state and this natural state continuously preserved throughout due to each population's strict adherence to their ancestral traditions on the dietary rules that had been passed on to them. As long as this state sustained Yin was good and fully operational, and each population's health was protected and its individual's good health was accordingly protected. Besides, with this substance in the body always, a deeply relaxing sleep every night, all reproductive functions including sexual potency and fertility, as well as memory are afforded naturally as Mother Nature's protection and further protects the body from all inflammation. I ascertain these as facts through my 6-7-8 years-long and continuing dietary study. If you are serious in maintaining your Yin fully operational at all times you can think of a truly disease-free life. Just as the Mother Nature provided! All free of charge! All of these and the modern so called degenerative diseases are caused by lack of this nutrient, that is, soluble fiber. I want you to understand and visualize that this watery substance called mucilage or soluble fiber is the very stuff that was always located inside the human body via the human's long held dietary habit throughout their entire evolutionary history and has become a permanent feature of human body physiology. This natural health protecting feature was partially disrupted since 1890's as I mentioned earlier. This is still in my opinion at this time.

Now say, Yin equals Water. Yin equals soluble fiber in water solution. This is the very **something viscous and elastic, or Yin Essence.** This may have been sought after by some healers in some populations around the globe as I explained above but was largely consumed hidden in their local traditional natural foods. I claim this to be the very food medicine that is responsible for protecting the human race from succumbing to diseases, and for continuing to thrive generation after generation until today. Now that you are made aware of this you can consciously look after this natural food medicine and include it in your diet to protect yourself from diseases.

If you find this dry word exercise tiring, try something real. Grab an avocado and a fruit knife. Slice it across the center and around the seed core. Twist to separate it into two halves. Dip your spoon into one and hand the other half to your companion. Yum! You can also try a persimmon. There are two kinds of persimmons: one is large with a pointy tip, which becomes edible only after when it got softened enough in late fall to winter; and the other called sweet persimmon is edible as soon as fully grown, usually in September to October. Avocado and persimmon, these two fruits are among my favorites. And add papaya, please! And some little raspberries, too, if you like! I believe all of these foods are relatively rich sources of soluble fiber and with individually different characteristics.

When I sat down with my whole history inclusive of my 6-7-8 years-old food study that I am still continuing appears coming recently to conclusion or as far as it might go, pictures start emerging in my mind where there was total darkness or ignorance. The main driving force or lack thereof in my health history seems to be dehydration, yes, truly dehydration. I now truly appreciate the phrase I used to say Yin Deficiency, or deficiency of Yin. Let me pause and declare, "It's dehydration that is at the bottom of all preventable diseases. It's so easy to prevent. Just give adequate nutrition! I even exclaimed "Sprezzatura!" "Ddang jipgo heieomchigida!" It's like swimming on the floor! So much pain over the years and years can be swept away in advance before anything comes to roost in your body. Now with this nutrient most troublesome health troubles can be stopped well in advance and prevented good. No more sickness! Here you have found the treasure of all the healers around the globe, including the ancient Egypt, have searched for.

But pause! For everything depends on your choice. Where your mind rests that will be your choice. Another pause! As I have commented earlier, the younger generations seem to have difficulty with high fiber foods. That's where my concern is. Young folks seem to like the polished rice and white bread. How are we to educate the young people against something they like? Like genies once out of the bottle, it's hard to contain them.

Apparent dehydration not understood by nutritional experts who c-l-i-n-g to, in my opinion, a faulty idea of hydration. In my opinion, "something slippery and sticky from the diet" is the essential precondition before proper hydration is achieved. This is our fate, if you will, so we'd better accept it.

My imagination once again is running back to the times when the earth was practically covered by tall grasses miles after miles and varied grass feeding animals roamed free or enterprising nomads rounded some of them up and became the herders, and others who found themselves on a fertile patch riverside found it profitable to farm and settled right down there. From this period on human diet has been largely predicated by seeds such as grass, grains, and beans. Human diet's fiber consumption may have peaked at this period, and as history marched on they came to build steady local dietary traditions under different cultures and religions. Even the world's some of the most isolated primitive tribes around the globe successfully maintained their dietary traditions that kept the populations healthy including their dental structure and maintenance as eminently reported by global trotting dentist researcher Dr. Weston A. Price in his rare gem of a book titled Nutrition and Physical Degeneration.

I might make a little confession here although I am fully aware that I am likely to be misjudged and misunderstood by people close to me including some of friends and family. Especially my own daughter might get consternated to learn that I have stopped brushing my teeth for years while living in her house. Because my mouth and teeth stay clean and free of any foul smell all the time, I

eventually got tired of brushing business and got rid of it. I cooked my own meals separately for my own purpose of living healthy and free of any disease or to minimize chances of any inflammatory pressures throughout my entire body, and beside I needed to deal with my own special diet so that I would go through symptom-free after I decided to discontinue my ENT prescribed medication. And I'm happy to report that everything is going well as I planned.

Now I can say that in my foods and lifestyle I have successfully duplicated what **Dr. Weston A. Price** found in some of the most isolated and primitive communities around the world. When I read the book years ago a question kept bugging myself was: "What was it specifically that allowed the people healthy and free of diseases so that I can copy them?" Now I know I must have successfully duplicated what is most critical in their diet. I am sure what it is now. It is soluble fiber, the very ultimate health food! This must have been well represented in whatever they might have eaten by scraping the land on top of what game and fish they could get, if any in the primitive environment they lived in. Therefore, there was pretty much of Mother Nature's hand in there.

On these scenes arrives modern era with beautiful (?) white flour complete in sacks ready to be baked and plenty of meat to go with. How can they resist? Our young people may be well educated but they are apparently not buying the high fiber value in nutrition and they are found in accelerated dehydration ahead of their seniors. This big discrepancy baffles the experts. They don't seem to recognize the dehydration occurring in front of their own eyes.

U.S. NEWS 12/04/2018
12 Million Pounds of Beef Now Under Recall Over Salmonella Risk
Nearly 250 people in 26 states have contracted salmonella poisoning, the USDA says.
By Sara Boboltz, Reporter, HuffPost
The United States Department of Agriculture on Tuesday announced an expanded nationwide beef recall due to new concerns over possible salmonella contamination.

Nearly 250 people in 26 states have fallen ill, the USDA's Food Safety and Inspection Service says. The agency fears more contaminated beef may be stored in Americans' freezers.

While most individuals who contract salmonella recover without treatment, the bacteria are particularly dangerous in children, the elderly and people with weakened immune systems. Symptoms develop between 12 to 72 hours after eating a contaminated substance and include diarrhea, abdominal cramps and fever. They usually last between four to seven days.

The affected products were packed on various dates between July 26 and Sept. 7 by JBS Tollerson, an Arizona-based beef processing plant that ships nationwide. The specific products subject to recall are stamped with "EST 267" within the USDA mark of inspection, the agency says.

A list of affected labels can be found on the USDA's website.

The salmonella scare comes shortly after a pre-Thanksgiving E. coli outbreak, which prompted the Centers for Disease Control and Prevention to tell Americans that they should throw away all romaine lettuce. Contaminated romaine has sickened 43 people in 12 states, the CDC says.

The lesson I got from my "good" leg: My right leg was spared or so I believed after a 1995 accident broke the tibia in my left leg. In an early morning, I was exercising walking along on the far-right side of a residential street in what was known as Korea Town in Los Angeles, pumping irons up and down in my both hands. I was hit by a car driving directly facing me head on. Its front bumper hit my left leg and I suffered a broken tibia. I was apparently spun around by the impact and was hit again at my right chest by the advancing car and suffered two chest ribs cracked. In September 2016, in a few months since moving back to California, and after 21 years of the accident, I wanted to find out some answers on my persistent walking difficulties that seemed to continue to deteriorate and had an x-ray taken out. The result as reported by the doctor appeared to be unremarkable to me. It said, "The sacroiliac (pelvis) joints are well preserved. There is moderate decrease in cartilage on the left side of hip joint and mild on the right side. Good for your age. Let me know if you would try physical therapy." After reading the report I failed to see the point of taking physical therapy and let it drop. Around that time and thereafter I could not walk as fast as I used to. In a couple of years, the problem got worse and worse so that my hips felt heavy like a rock and my right leg was dangled at the hip, the knee and the ankle, at those three joints at the same time while I dragged myself along to walk. I eventually got resigned to the situation and accepted my right leg would be a cripple for the rest of my life. But it was not to be!? I wasn't sure but I looked for eventual healing to take place. The diet I have been using with plenty of mucilage rich foods for years since 2012 apparently began helping reverse the dehydration that was going on in my body, and now started to be positively hydrating my body day by day, which I have been monitoring. Around the end of May, 2018, I had a memorable event that told me that the hydration that has been progressing in my body has finally reached the distal end of my guts, cured the chronic dehydration there, also known as constipation and promises to keep the place hydrated all the time thereafter. During the next week or two my body was giving me mysterious signals on my right leg as if trying to switch gears. For a day or two the joints on my right leg felt very light as if I could walk just as if normal and the weight I felt at my low back was definitely lightening. Promptly after my Foot Great Yin Organ the Spleen (The Digestive Tract, in my understanding) was taken care of, my body was turning its eyes on mending my legs. I knew that was what was happening as the Eastern Medicine teaches that the Spleen governs both arms and legs and figured that more walking wouldn't hurt me now. In early November 2017 I doubled my daily walking into one hour each in the morning and afternoon. I also reversed the slowing of my recent walking speed and started walking faster to keep the house pet dog Amalia on a trot. This too was also a change from recent habit. All in all I'm doing great, energized and not tired at all as I used to be all the time in the several recent years. It's dawning on me now that finally resolving the lagging dehydration/ Yin Deficiency must be the explanation for it. Is that truly what I think it is? I feel I'm almost in a living dream. Well, Yin Deficiency may be in receding. But I must be still in my twilight zone of life and when I take a seat I kind of slump into it. I have to see how it's going to work out. Anyway, I look forward to living some more years like this if I'm allowed to do so. But my euphoria didn't last long. I finally admitted barely after a couple of weeks I was pushing myself too hard and too fast. I was forced to slow down and cut back on walking. On a reduced schedule I start feeling better, and I'm going to be patient and look for the long haul. As of now 11/11/19, nearly 3 years ago as I reported earlier, my right leg dangles at 3 joints at different times, right or wrong, the cause this time may be associated with the 1995 auto accident, or otherwise nothing else is in my mind. I tend to imagine the rapid twirl somehow may have caused a sufficient impact to cause the damage I am experiencing now. I have never heard of the kind, but that is the only thing I can think of at this time. After all these theories seemingly unable to explain the malady in my right leg now I tend to ascribe it to an hiking accident in which I slipped in the first snow on November First, probably in the year 2007. I had first guessed the childhood malnutrition was the cause, but I eventually ruled that out. Now on 2/17/20 I am firmly convinced that it must be "a big toe malady caused by twisting it out of its proper joint sideways, although I have never heard of a trouble like this but I have suffered long enough to know what it is by now. I'll call it "Displaced Big Toe Syndrome," which has already made me very difficult to walk. I realize now it's too late to help. I ruled out surgery at my age. So,

I am resigned to suffer its eventuality whatever it may end up with. I hope my readers will be wiser and not to neglect their big toe if anything happened to it.

I Started My Study While Living Temporarily in Korea

Back in the years 2010-14 while I stayed in Korea temporarily to care for my mother, I chose to live in a rural area where I had free access to some chestnuts and persimmons in the fall. All the young folks who grew up in the countryside chose to move to the cities where jobs are with their growing families, so the occasional old and idle transplants like me found plenty of housing and accommodations in the countryside. The chestnuts were not only delicious but also noted for their anti-inflammatory action, translated food medicine, I found out. I was also given free access to several small persimmon trees bearing puny little fruit called pickling persimmons and standing in steep hills. I used to love as a child the little ones pickled in brine and eaten as a cold winter night snack. During the last 20 to 30 years, however, the large so called king persimmons which used to be rare were widely propagated and caused the market for the smaller ones, that is, pickling persimmons collapse. So now it didn't make sense for the local growers to hire workers to harvest them and instead they offered them to me free. I accepted them gratefully and made a daily hike in lieu of my walking routine with a long bamboo pole in hands in December through January picked a few every day. I ate them later when they got softened enough. This gave me fun, exercise as well as good food so it was a win-win for me. I enjoyed the experience wholeheartedly. Thank you!

While enjoying the routine I began entertaining a notion of something unusual. I began to see the softened persimmons at a different angle from the traditional way. Most Koreans saw a softened persimmon as an aid to stop diarrhea. Now I have learned to see it as a gel rich source food, in other words, a Yin food. Perhaps, an excuse to eat more of the yummy little ones without diarrhea!? Anyway, because I was a California licensed acupuncturist and idled in part by having left the state I wished to find something worthwhile to do while staying in Korea. And on the one hand I have been going through a sort of personal transition in life entering 70's in age. Maybe I'll study my own health experiences I'll be going through these years. My childhood history of malnutrition was considered the cause of Yin Deficiency and emaciation into the adulthood. For nearly two decades I was one of the aggressive and steady hikers around Mt. Wilson in the Angeles National Forest, but I was curious about my legs having no muscular bulges, and I was silently blaming the fact on my childhood malnutrition.

And, therefore, I was strongly interested in studying the so-called Yin Deficiency Syndrome, and with several symptoms attributed to it. To my great surprise and satisfaction, in just a few months of starting my dietary addition of mucilage rich foods such as flax seeds, chia seeds, ma and softened persimmons, and non-bitter so called "sweet persimmons" in various combinations, and perhaps including quite a few of chests nuts as well. I began to notice my lower legs bulging with muscular balls I have so long missed. I was so ecstatic, so flabbergasted and happy to see them having suddenly appeared in my flesh in my early 70's of age. This was one of the first three fantastic changes I experienced on my body. The other two were good night's sleep every night, which I missed in most of my earlier years, and the early morning experience of waking up with my man sticking up like when I was a boy, again in my early 70's. Nowadays I take naps as well as night sleep. I have never struggled to fall asleep either in my night sleep or in my daily nap. As soon as I settle down in bed I fall asleep. It's like automatic, or as one may call it "natural."

I felt as if the fiber in nutrition may have served as some kind of core fiber of the musculature development and strength both on the legs as well as the small organ between my legs. And over the months and years my once emaciated legs now carry fully well-developed musculature, apparently from the years of long distance walking done back in my 40's through 50's. Do muscles appear after sleeping 20 to 30 years? I find it hard to believe but that is exactly what I see on my legs although my mobility through my 70's was largely limited or struggling to walk for about a year or so. But now I feel a slight hint of getting eased in walking. I'm not sure but I'm cautiously optimistic, hopeful in the last year or so. Therefore, I must give credit to my consuming of mucilage rich foods somehow responsible for them. Thanks to my mucilage rich foods helping hydration my lifelong emaciation has been replaced by fully fleshed out musculature throughout the body.

And currently a large portion of population of our society is woefully unmet in this basic requirement of life, I suspect, and as its consequence, suffer a stampede of chronic illnesses such as insomnia, so called erectile dysfunction, obesity, type 2 diabetes, dementia, arthritis and some nerve damaging degenerative diseases such as Parkinson's, Altzheimer's, etc. These ailments were traditionally considered due to Yin Deficiency and were relatively rare except in old ages, but now they are widespread and into the younger age groups as well. Sleeplessness was exclusively old folks' problem. Not anymore! In recent years such mundane things as sleep depravedness, erectile failure, constipation, etc., have become parts of the national epidemics. People are clamoring for help. During the several years following the year 2000, when I got my acupuncture license, I got familiarized that among the menopausal women patients the roasted flax seeds were popular "food medicine" known for the reputation for allegedly relieving or lessening certain of their menopausal complaints. Now I realize that flax seeds are one of the gel rich Yin foods, and as such would do well to protect the women if they included them in their regular diet. I believe there is certain disconnect in people's understanding in nature and health in the United States. People largely look up to medical care and health insurance because that is what is intensely promoted by the interest groups, and there is little interest in old fashioned self-care and prevention. I believe the fiber's long term health protecting roles are currently sometimes discussed as improving health and named as functional health food or even as nutri-ceutical (a recently coined new word), but no one even suspect our loss of natural health protection from disease and pain due to the loss of people's memory on their ancestral traditional diet.

I think we need a solid public health education based on self-care according to the proper traditional nutrition. Now you see why this approach can take us a long distance because the most basic and universal cause for disease is dehydration and we can minimize that nationally, and as many as all individuals in America now possess their personal power to free themselves from all those diseases by the individuals' conscious action of proper nutrition. By popularizing this idea we can make a great contribution toward public health as well as your own health and freedom from pain. Just mind your nutrition on daily basis according to this traditional diet. That would be your true whole healthcare for life, guaranteed by the Mother Nature's natural protection.

Consider as our 2020 presidential election campaigns get heated some leading democratic leaders call for national free health care. This is apparently because they listened to the peoples' predicaments clamoring for health care, felt sympathetic to them and try to represent them. It's noble in their intentions but factually I believe they may be misguided due to what I know is true. But it's not their fault that they are misguided because I feel everybody else seems to be misguided. Do scientists know? They might, but I am not in position to know, yes or no.

I remember reading someone a few years ago on the internet, saying: "There is no pure water inside the body. The moment you drink a cup of water as it goes down washes the walls of the esophagus and when it reaches the stomach it is no longer the pure water. It contains something in it." I do not recall any further details, but it might be like "food residues or even some mucus" or something like that. I believe the writer was a biochemist. So, if this was a Western practitioner's typical expectation I see a picture of pretty healthy people, who are at least potentially well hydrated, for there is a hint apparently of some generic "viscous molecules." But this modicum of "viscous molecules" is no longer guaranteed in the modern American diet. Saliva is a given to most people, but some in America have trouble producing saliva in their mouths. The only reason that they cannot produce saliva that I know of is the lack of "viscous molecules" in the diet. Plenty are found in bran of grains such as wheat, barley, rice, oats and spelt, and in most fruits and vegetables. It's a myth to me how anybody can eat foods and end up not absorbing any "viscous molecules." But it's apparently happening in America creating an epidemic of degenerative diseases. As far as I know most degenerative diseases will not occur as long as plenty of "viscous molecules" are absorbed from soluble fiber rich foods in the diet. Without some "viscous molecules" in the guts, the body cannot beneficially access water, and in this body if water was drunk, it will not going to nourish the body. I can't offer a scientific proof but I offer my testimony of personal truth. I have told you how my body "truly hydrating" only after consuming "viscous molecules" everyday continuously for 6 full years and I still continue as long as I may live. This is the story of true hydration as I personally experienced. No conjugated "viscous molecules" no hydration possible! Period! Well, at this point this may be just an opinion of mine and perhaps an enigma to many others. But I am sure you can personally verify this truth by trying the very diet I recommend.

In my opinion again, there are two tracts eventually leading to a degenerative condition. One is the ancient one, that is, diabetes, traditionally known as rich men's/women's disease, specifically caused by nutritional excess, that is, too much glucose consumed or metabolized. All other instances of degenerative diseases occur, in my opinion, due to dehydration by a special kind of modern nutritional deficiency. Yes, an unusual kind of nutritional deficiency, of which origin may trace back to the year 1890 or later, by inventing grain polishing machines first time in history and polishing off the grains to make them "more palatable" according to some people's misconceived ideas.

Contrary to popular misconception, dehydration is caused by the

loss of the essential nutrients previously described as "viscous molecules," as a direct consequence of use of the grain polishing machines. I say these "viscous molecules" must be recognized as a critical conjugated partner of water that would make proper hydration of body possible. At this point I need to make a decision on my use of the term "viscous molecules." I want to use its generic substitute like mucilage or soluble fiber as interchangeable. Thus, with some mucilage or soluble fiber mixed with drunk water recognized as essential nutrients, that would have helped prevent dehydration from happening in the first place, and later any degenerative diseases. The full implication of proper hydration is potentially preventing all inflammatory diseases. It is my sincere hope, therefore, to see the day that this hydration enigma eventually taken up and cleared up by scientists and health professionals and its full public health implications such as consumers' self-care potentials toward cultivating their own disease prevention and self-health maintenance care following the dietary recommendations fully discussed in all entry level physiology texts published.

And water is the most important nutrient for long term health maintenance, strength and beauty of the skin and musculature as well as the brain itself and memory, and ultimately the freedom from diseases. As we get older, body's ability to retain water may decrease and we become susceptible to some chronic diseases, which may torment our senior years depriving us of comfort and relaxation we deserve in our twilight years. I feel so distressed to hear some of those people plead to be allowed to end their lives because they feel they are trapped in endless pain and lost hope of ending the pain ever. If you feel you are trapped in pain, it may not be easy to recommend where to act. In my opinion, pain is caused ultimately as the inflammatory pressure tips the scale against the body's self-defense forces. Therefore, my ultimate position in pain-free living is reducing the inflammatory pressure by choosing the foods, what to eat, and what not! The diet I pursue personally and recommend interested readers is geared to minimize the inflammatory pressures and help strengthen the body's defensive forces. The following section is designed to guide my readers in disease-free and pain-free living.

My Journey Seeking the Ultimate Truth Found Mucilage Providing
The Core Biological Corridor for Lifetime Freedom from Diseases;
The Rest is Own Self-Care on Nutrients and Lifestyle Choices;
It Thus Restores "Self-Care," the CHIEF OF HUMAN HEALTH

CARE.

In the very beginning of life on earth a bacterium created mucilage, scientists say. From this one bacterium many mucilage creating bacteria multiplied in succession creating a class of mucilage creating soil bacteria and eventually covering much of the land areas of the earth. The various emerging plant forms benefitted from the moisture holding soil bacteria and readily adopted mucilage as part of their organic body structure. The mucilage inside the plants helped them grow larger and stronger and eventually all plants adopted mucilage creating trait as their own as they are known today. In my opinion, the mucilage was readily adopted by animals as they emerged and began eating plants as their food. The ability to hold an amount of water as part of their bodies was a great advantage for the animals, and eventually the physiological mechanism to use the mucilage regularly came to be built in as we see today. All later developed higher animal species, hominids and eventually homo inherited the same trait, and this is what I believe happened to all human ancestors. The few most striking points in this reconstructive story are: first, water is the single most important essential resource required for all life forms both plants and animals including humans, which is freely available from nature; Water is the major component of our body cells, tissues and all organs and systems, and roughly 70%-80% of our body's weight is composed in water; In my opinion, however, there is hardly any other human being who understands precisely the intimate relationship which water commands in relation with the integrity of human body's physiology. I am neither a physiologist nor even a biologist. But as an intimate observer of my own body I lived through and experienced changes that occurred to my body over the last 6-7-8 years by now, running a personal dietary experiment, and proved my own theory, to my complete personal satisfaction, that a human body is designed to protect its integrity while living in nature throughout one's lifetime and free from diseases by the force of water's inherent anti-inflammatory action when it is properly interfaced by the layer of mucilage facilitating proper and effective hydration to occur with the intimate cell structures of human body. Without this proper interface existing, a proper and effective hydration fails to occur to human body, in my opinion, regardless how much water is, or how often, drunk and automatically leads to dehydration and disease. In my opinion dehydration is the most major cause of various human chronic diseases. The sinus problem I have had nearly 50 years, long without any clue about how to get rid of it, I finally defeated it single-handedly by discovering and utilizing my body's own ancient built-in natural technology, completely demolished it molecule by molecule. And guess what, I think I discovered in the process my body's own ability to dismantle the disease-causing mechanism itself and turn it around to make it health-building, instead. **The key to turn on or turn off in my body's mechanism was the hydration, yes, true hydration, for there is such a thing as false hydration that is passed out as if it is true in our society including the very professionals who should know better.** This is a tricky question right now because our society is going through a change from the long held traditional diet which seems to be practically abandoned by our younger people and there is no societal agreement on a healthful, sound and agreeable established version is in place yet, in my opinion.

My point is that our proper diet must include the traditional mucilage rich foods for the very reason that the mucilage would give immunity to diseases and help people stay healthy throughout.

Let's not obfuscate this fact and make sure this fact is well understood among the people of our communities. I respectfully insist that one of the goals in our proper diet should be building immunity and I say that the only way to do so is to eat a plenty of mucilage rich foods throughout the day, preferably at least two meals per day so that next time you drink water it will find enough mucilage on the walls of your esophagus and gets mixed-in with it, for this is the only possible way a true, proper, and effective hydration is allowed to happen in your body, and that is the very key to turn off the disease causing mechanism of your body, and instead turn on the health and immunity building key. *I thought that was what you would want. Wasn't that right?*

And I also want to point out that all Yin organs and meridians are the ones that accept directly from the nature and process essential supplies for life such as water, food, and air into forms body can profitably utilize, or metabolize. This is all taken care of, as I said, by our bodies' main work horse epithelial cells strategically placed around body. If this was allowed to happen naturally the human race is predicated to survive indefinitely without much of currently debilitating diseases. It is not accident that most of the cancers, up to 90 percent, occur in epithelial cells. Such diseases occur only because the natural processes that provided over millennia are now compromised, I believe, by deficiency in nutrition, that is, soluble fiber dissolved in water is largely missing in the affected populations.

Therefore, I am closing this preface by quoting from an article from encyclopedia.com as accessed on 12/17/17, which seems to largely congruent to what I presented so far. But I am deeply concerned about the direction we may be heading.

FIBER, DIETARY. In 1972 British physician Hugh Trowell defined fiber as "that portion of the food which is derived from cellular walls of plants which is digested very poorly by human beings" (*Revue Europeenne d'Etudes Cliniques et Biologiques*). Most of the current interest in dietary fiber stems from the efforts of Trowell and other researchers in the 1960s and 1970s to examine the differences in disease patterns between populations consuming high in refined foods (typical of developed countries) and populations consuming high in unrefined foods (typical of less developed or undeveloped countries). Populations of a higher intake of unrefined food, and thus a higher intake of dietary fiber, had lower risk of chronic diseases, such as heart disease, intestinal cancers, and gastrointestinal disorders, as compared to populations consuming highly refined, low fiber diets. These observations stimulated a large number of research studies and, *while the ability of fiber to prevent chronic disease is difficult to prove, the data gathered since 1960s strongly supports the importance of dietary fiber for the health of the gastrointestinal tract and thus its importance in the general diet.*

As you read above, the populations in developed countries tend to consume high in refined foods, and although those in undeveloped or underdeveloped countries currently consume high in unrefined foods but in the long run as they are trying to modernize their economies they are more than likely to follow their developed cousins' models and lose track of some of their cultural heritage in living close to the earth and consuming relatively large amount of their diet from locally produced plant sourced foods. A higher population growth and resulting urbanization in the now less developed countries will likely further erode their reliance on their traditional diet and lifestyle. For this seems to be our likely future it raises my concern.

In summary, I hereby state clearly as result of my successful experiment, and claim the right to say that I proved, that every human being has inherited biological protection from disease and pain due to the disease, by the proper habitual daily ingestion of mucilage rich foods such as described in this book, because I was just one individual of the humanity, who must have inherited this internal protective mechanism from the ultimate ancestors, from whom all currently living human individuals must have descended.

The mucilage was probably richly contained in all parts of plants human ancestors chose to pick such as leaves, stems, flowers, fruits, seeds, roots, vines, and tubers, or any edible parts such as the tender and richly juicy inner barks of certain plants and trees. When the evolution of humanity reached tribal societies, the elders probably prescribed what they considered essential for their survival and prosperity, which probably in myriads of ethnic groups in the long lines of successions, handed down eventually something described as traditional ethnic food. I trust that the traditional ethnic food was largely successful in protecting and supporting the integrity of the built-in natural health maintenance system in human physiology as I describe in this book, and thus we inherit the system in our bodies. But I believe the events following the invention and introduction of milling machines in the 1890's still poses serious challenges to us today. The challenges we face today haven't met appropriate responses, yet. An individual human being stands on the foundation of food security and health maintenance. When a person stands with his/her own feet firmly on this foundation, he/she can go out, work and compete freely, and provide the best for his/her family. Therefore, the lack of health security hampers the individual seriously. We all heard the large crowds of people screaming for healthcare in recent democratic election campaigns. **It's about time we told them that they already have a built-in health protection system in their individual bodies by Mother Nature's grace, and how to effectively activate the system for their own individual bodies by proper nutrition. – Yes, only by using proper nutrition daily, every day of your life. That will give you free healthcare by Mother Nature, better than anything you've heard of.**

<u>Importance of Public Education on Individual Health Maintenance</u>

I suppose the human survival and prosperity greatly depends on individual health maintenance and wellbeing. As modern society diversifies individuals tend to get lost in their traditional self-health care practice and we need to educate them the potentials of what they can contribute to maintain and improve their own health. **I urge my readers to personally replicate my food only healing experiment. If you are under a doctor's care you should consult your doctor and work with his or her approval.**

On the other hand, I ask all of my readers to join me in personally replicating my food only self-healing experiment, and after a few to several years, depending on your age and your current health conditions, hopefully as well as assuredly, each of you having vanquished your chronic diseases and any of the resulting pain, I believe and trust the strength of the Mother Nature's hand in protecting humanity from succumbing to the vagaries of existence on earth through the long evolutionary period will continue to

strengthen us and eventually step up enough pressure to move the now silent scientific community to admit the human body's self-healing mechanism built-in by Mother Nature into all of their textbooks of Human Anatomy and Physiology. If and when this happened these books as the basis of all manner of public health education in the primary and the secondary schools as well as for the general public, which I trust will greatly contribute to the better health of the people of this country and beyond.

Chapter 3

WHAT DOES YIN-YANG REALLY MEAN PHYSICALLY?

Anything you can do, or dream you can, begin it.
Boldness has genius, power, and magic in it."
— Goethe

I tested the selected foods personally on my body by eating them as part of the meals most every day. Some of these foods were considered in the local culture like a food medicine, or carry fancy folklore. I included several other foods that are not so well known but share the similar characteristics. This adventure spread over now fully 6-7-8-9 and 10 years, since March 2012 until this day 5/26/20, gave me confidence that I found the main food item that is probably responsible for having kept humans alive over the millennia, and which is responsible to carry me in tandem through my life trouble-free. This is my lifetime commitment.

This is a large claim. I realize that and mean it. Since I had closed my young practice in Acupuncture and Oriental Medicine in Glendale, California after just 5 years and left at the end of February 2006, I felt my career was not finished but interrupted. I had always wanted to get back but there were two hurdles. One that was obvious was lack of finances. The other was invisible one and only known to my Self, which was, to write this book and get it published. Then and only then I would feel ready to open an office. Unfortunately for my career, it took me so long to finish this book. Now this is the book that I have been dreaming about writing. I was always thinking and working on it like a hen sitting on her eggs constantly and keeping them warm.

(I want to make a special note here, that I had been distressed by suffering urinary urgency and inability to hold for about 5 years between my 70th and 74th years, which I would call it as my broken water controlling system. As I got healed of this distressing condition within a couple of years of starting the mucilage rich foods since my mid-74th year I came to realize slowly progressively more positively that the urinary must be only a part of a larger and integral self-maintenance system, which I may call an old-fashioned word constitution. The word constitution in my Merriam Webster's Collegiate Dictionary is defined "2a the physical makeup of the individual comprising inherited qualities modified by environment." This is a body of a self-standing, -defending, -maintaining, -correcting (or –healing) integral individual entity, that is free-roaming in nature. This body is not ever-living or omnipotent. But the body has developed an incredibly sophisticated self-perpetuating life-support system out of having eaten seemingly simple things available in nature that boggles my mind. It certainly demands my utmost respect. In a nod of my respect I would capitalize the word the Constitution. Further discussions will follow later.)

In the Yin-Yang Concept Balance Is the Key

Now that I have established with you that water is indeed one of the primary essential nutrients, I'm ready to go back to my discussion of Yin Food and Yang Food. As I said in the beginning the ultimate Yin Food is water and Yang Food is any or all of the calorie-producing foods such as proteins, carbohydrates and lipids. As I also said in the beginning, neither Yin nor Yang alone is absolutely good or bad. To be good the both sides must work together and compromise with each other, and they had to be fairly well balanced against each other. When that happens and persists you get great health. It is important to remember we need to retain this balanced state of health.

So let's place the Yin-Yang and associated concepts in two contrasting columns. The words from a totally different culture may sound weird, but I assure you that the idea is pretty sensible and you can relate to it. So please have some patience and note that the Yin/Water on the left is anti-inflammatory by its nature, while Yang/Fire on the right is potentially pro-inflammatory when in excess. And this is the basic set up of the relationship between the two.

Anti-inflammatory Yin (Water/fiber)	Pro-Inflammatory Yang (Fire/Fuel)
• Non-calorie Producing Food	• Calorie Producing Food
• Water/Fiber or mucilage	• Carbohydrates, Lipids, Proteins broken down to glucose

<table>
<tr><td>

- Cooling, moistening influence
- Slows down digestion, Reduces inflammation

</td><td>

- Warming influence, partly depriving moisture
- Promotes digestion, growth, reproduction and may promote inflammation if in excess

</td></tr>
</table>

Table 2. Yin-Yang Model Helps Demystify Complex Health Choices into Stark Contrasts

As you see in the columns above, Yin/Water reduces inflammation, while Yang/Fire promotes it, working diametrically opposite way. In this particular relationship as presented above, Yin and Yang each gives and takes, while moderating the forces of each other. As long as both sides stay operating this way the body is in a more or less balanced state and can go on like that indefinitely.

Let's Scrutinize Left Column First

The column on the left represents the forces of Yin/Water, or Water/Fiber, or mucilage, and it has cooling energy. Please note that Yin/Water is not just pure water, but rather the kind of water that we come to absorb from our food plants as we eat them, although I am not necessarily exclude other types of water. This water is part of a living plant. Naturally, this water holds onto moisture and resists drying. Although much of the weight should be pure water, it has been incorporated into organic structure of the plant and as such may be called organic water with unique qualities. To our everyday experiences, the juices when rubbed between the fingers feel slippery or elastic, and a little later when they get a bit dry they become sticky or viscous. Thus the

Let's Examine the Right Column Now

The very important balance must be achieved between non-calorie producing food and calorie producing food, in other words, between water/fiber against the ultimate amount of glucose. If more glucose is produced than body can use profitably, then the excess calories will eventually and necessarily turn inflammatory. Warming influence supports activities, and also possible to deprive moisture under circumstances. Today's exploding obesity and type-2 diabetes, the two major phenomena resulting from the excess consumption on the calorie producing food showcase how challenging it is for us to eat moderately all the time. Even if we individuals tried to limit we tend to gain weight incrementally little by little and eventually many of us reach a point visco-elastic qualities of these liquids provide can be very useful when absorbed into our bodies as we will see. We probably need to eat a wide spectrum of them in our food. This is the Yin food that protects our body from inflammation. of no return. In recent months, I realized I got myself nearly trapped there, and learned to see it as a phenomenon of inflammation, and by fighting it as such now I begin to get loosened. I think this is a good strategy, and will stay that way.

Valuable Interface Shield with Mucus

The Yin food, as I talked about above, or mucilage rich food, in our diet is essential in fighting inflammation and disease and keeping you healthy. While there are many ways the mucilage rich food helps the most important and far-reaching way would be that it strengthens the body's Yin System over time. By eating such food regularly you can help maintain your strong Constitution.

Although the details on how body does it exactly are not well known, I want to explore it and try to offer some understandings. In the Eastern Medicine six Yang Organs-and-Meridians, and six corresponding Yin Organs-and-Meridians are recognized. But I intend to discuss briefly here only about the Yin Organs-and-Meridians as they are relevant on how to strengthen the Yin System and keep it that way.

The Meridians are also known as channels, channeling Qi throughout the body. Of the six Yin channels three of them run through the upper extremities, and they are 1) Greater/Tai Yin Lung Channel, 2) Lesser/Shao Yin Heart Channel, and 3) Reverting/Jue Yin Pericardium Channel.

Other three of them run through the lower extremities, and they are 1) Greater/Tai Yin Spleen Channel, 2) Lesser/Shao Yin Kidney Channel, and 3) Reverting/Jue Yin Liver Channel. Further channel trajectory is out of scope of this book. Although how acupuncture works is not fully known scientifically it is undeniably practically useful, and I happen to notice, that all of the organs associated Yin channels listed above are served by epithelial cells that form barrier protecting the body's interior environment from the exterior environment of the nature.

The most prominent one of those channels by far is known as Foot Greater Yin of Spleen, which is often taken as roughly equivalent to digestive tract in the Western Medicine. Imagine as if you go through this 27 feet long tunnel-like region of your body as a tourist in a micro-miniature submersible vehicle in the size of a small imaginary water bug that would move freely through the thick or thin at times sheets of mucus, yes, mucus, or substances scientifically known as glycoproteins produced and released by the goblet cells lining the tract. I mean just visualize that every time you eat or drink something, especially when a large amount of food is eaten the whole gut is activated churning and churning. When there is some fatty food coming down the chute the gallbladder immediately squeezes out some bile into the duct toward the duodenum, which will help break down and emulsify the fat ready to be absorbed. When liver manufactures bile, it packages toxins in bile salts separated from the body along with the bile, and sends it down the guts and, if everything worked as it should, the underlying epithelial cells lining the guts will readily release some of its mucous membrane mass just in time to capture the toxins in bile salts, wrap them up with the stool tight and secure to be excreted out of the body. This is a natural process body has learned to get rid of the toxins it had to process and render itself harmless over the eons of evolutionary progress, which allowed us to survive this far. This process will go on and on day after day, year after year, like a clockwork indefinitely, only under one condition: that body will be given the resources at its disposal, that is, the nutrition of glycoproteins, or the sticky and slippery substances that make up the mucus and plenty of water to be part of it, for 95% of the intestinal sheets of mucus consists of water. The total amount of mucus released in a 24-hour period is staggering. Some sources say about 10 liters per day, although much of this is reabsorbed, and about 10% of it is wasted and excreted out of the body with the stool. The water in the mucus is where the nutrients are dissolved and held suspended until absorbed. How important that role alone is! Remember body cannot hold so much water in the guts or elsewhere without the partnership of mucus, or its viscoelastic substances, that is, in other words, glycoproteins.

I briefly highlighted above only one of the roles mucus plays in the guts. I think our general opinion on mucus is, if not disgusted, generally dismissive at best and we have no inkling about how important it is for our life and health. It is time to begin to recognize the importance of the strategic partnership of water and viscoelastic substances to form mucus in our body. Some of the mucus found in the intestinal tract is the living matter as the extension of the mucous membrane tissues of the epithelial cells. The mass of such mucus is humongous as noted in the brief quotation cited below. There are also some layers of mucus detached from the underlying cells but still hanging around in the area. You would be surprised to hear that some immunity cells live inside the mucus layers hiding to trap any unsuspecting bacteria, virus or toxins before they try to invade the body. I am greatly intrigued that these mucous layers made of water and viscoelastic substances may also work as a protective interface shield strategically placed just between the interior and the exterior, or between the living body tissues and the exterior environment of the nature, and as such there may be other multiple aspects exerting influences on the inflammatory pressures we go through daily, for example, as I feel in my body as I get older. I will pursue these aspects further later.

As I said earlier, the Spleen (**Note:** I consider this Eastern Medicine term is largely equivalent to the Digestive Tract of the Western Medicine.) is the most prominent one of the Yin Organs-and-Meridians as the Greater/Tai Yin of the Foot. The next prominent Yin Organ-and-Meridian is of the Lungs. Lungs and the rest of the respiratory tract are also serviced by epithelial cells and the surface areas are covered by mucus released by the underlying mucous membrane cells. The mucus consists of water and viscous-elastic substances, which, in my view, represent the nature's simple but most appropriate biotechnology of self-protection. Without this mucus we cannot breathe. Without this mucus properly supplied and circulated we can neither smell nor taste food. And I can say the same thing about our ears and hearing. The mucus in the mouth is in the form of saliva, and in other places of the body, it may be more appropriate to call it simply fluids. Without saliva, or body fluids, we cannot chew, swallow or eat food. Do you realize how far-reaching impact mucus has in our lives? It is a mundane everyday thing we never think about unless you lost its proper function of it. Yes, there are some elderly people who lost ability to produce saliva in their mouths. Scientists say the mucus is produced by the goblet cells and mucus cells of the epithelia. But where does the raw material of the mucus ultimately come from? It must be the diet. But diet changes over time and cultures. Especially with industrialization and urbanization the changes have been dramatic, which are still going on. Conscientious parents encourage their children to eat more vegetables, but often it is an unwinnable struggle. Is it possible on individuals who eat not enough vegetables can be of short supply of what I call slippery and sticky substances to produce enough mucus for the mucus membranes for their bodies? A resounding yes should be the logical answer, and especially so with the young school age children???!!!

I want to draw your attention now back to the article I quoted above: *Water as an Essential Nutrient.* Under the subhead *"Water as a lubricant and shock absorber,"* where it says:

Water, in combination with viscous molecules, forms lubricating fluids for joints; for saliva, gastric and intestinal mucus secretion in the digestive tract; for mucus secretion in the airways in the respiratory system; and for mucus secretion in the genitourinary tract.

By maintaining the cellular shape, water also acts as a shock absorber during walking or running. This function is important for the brain and the spinal cord, and is particularly important for the fetus, who is protected by a water cushion.

The viscoelastic water/fluid provides lubrication to various organs and systems in the body, where it is strategically needed in the communication with the nature for survival, that is, exchange of air, introduction of food and water, excretion of wastes, and reproduction of an offspring and all those associated organs function normally as intended.

Just for a few examples; a) On the skeletal joints lubricating fluids facilitate free movement, prevent stress and pain; b) Healthy people may not realize how valuable saliva is. Saliva not only moistens mouth and lips but also protects structures in the mouth, teeth such as gums, tongue, and cheeks from infection. People with parched mouth with little saliva production having trouble in chewing and swallowing food need amplified saliva production. Drinking plain water alone doesn't help these people. This condition offers stark proof that drinking water alone fails to hydrate human body. As I explained earlier, for proper hydration to take place in human body we need plenty of the viscoelastic substances dissolved in the water on the walls of esophagus supplied from our regular dietary habit of consuming plenty of mucilage or soluble fiber daily. Because the people consume little soluble fiber their bodies are deprived in Yin, and therefore, no effective hydration takes place in their bodies. The only way to help these people is to let them eat Yin food with mucilage in it. And a plenty of it! Period! There is no other way around it.

All of these activities involve hazards such as abrasion, introduction of foreign matter, invasion of bacteria, etc. The mucous layers covering the digestive, respiratory, as well as the genitourinary tracts provide a protective shell for the body's front line agents, namely the epithelial cells, working to process the passing materials while protecting the underlying structures. Viscous water also works to maintain stability of the floating structures such as brain, spinal column and the developing fetus.

These are just a few of the larger organs and systems served by the epithelial type cells and tissues. Here are more details. **"Although firmly attached to underlying structures, an epithelium always has free surface exposed to the environment or to some internal chamber or passageway. Epithelia are dominated by cells in close contact with one another, and there are few extracellular materials. This tissue** type covers every exposed body surface, and also lines the digestive, respiratory, reproductive, and urinary tracts, internal passageways that communicate with outside world. Epithelia also surround internal cavities, lining the chest cavity, the fluid-filled chambers in the brain, eye and inner ear, and the inner surfaces of blood vessels and the heart."[1] Those epithelial cells are designed to carry out life-supporting activities while protecting the internal environment from potential harms from outside.

[1] Martini, Frederic, PhD, Fundamentals of Anatomy and Physiology, Prentice-Hall International Editions, ©1989 by Prentice-Hall Inc., A Division of Simon & Schuster, Englewood Cliffs, New Jersey 07632

Humans Can't Afford to Go Astray Far from Mucilage Rich Diet Our Bodies Are Built and Fixed to Work That Way Trouble-Free

Now let's take a look at how peoples' attitudes and preferences toward our essential foods necessary for our survival have drastically changed in recent decades. Most prominent changes are that the Western industrialized societies are leading the world in the increased meat consumption, and also decreased vegetable/roughage consumption at the same time. I believe these changes in diet multiplied calorie consumption into far excess above normal balanced human dietary regimes and have already generated serious public health issues such as widespread obesity, again widespread type 2 diabetes and other degenerative diseases.

I also hear that some people suffer from chronic pain so severe and hopeless to end that they want their doctors to end their lives. In my view pain is a function of inflammation and the inflammatory pressure of the whole body. To reduce inflammatory pressure one should consider dietary changes to reduce calorie consumption and lifestyle habits such as more exercise. I hear others while trying to cope with their pain got addiction to opioids, which is also nearly impossible to shake off for good, and that is the main problem. And I also hear many of these people are young athletics who got trapped in it while trying to cope with their sports injuries. I am at a loss in how to help this case. Traditionally only in limited hospice situation narcotics were allowed to treat pain. Otherwise, one should be extremely cautious of any contact with narcotics. I also hear some elderly who lost their memory completely and are shut in an institution away from their loved ones. It tears my heart when I read these stories. Many of these cases sound like fairly advanced.

Prevention is the best strategy. However, as long as you continue the mucilage rich foods I describe, I strongly believe that you will eventually be free from all diseases and pain in the next 5 to 10 years,

in case of an adult and with children probably sooner. Unknown to you and many others, I am telling you that we human beings are genetically protected by Mother Nature through the means of proper diet so that our bodies shall be free from disease. I believe that's how the humanity has survived so far. Therefore, prevention offers the best choice. Always choose prevention.

As I have already stated clearly, my main strategy for health is prevention. The humanity is lucky to have an effective nature-endowed lifetime healthcare system but in recent decades especially those of us living in so called industrialized and developed regions of the world are largely distracted from the traditional diet and for that reason we are losing our natural healthcare benefits to be provided via true hydration, for the true hydration is only achieved when we take enough mucilage, or soluble fiber, or visco-elastic substances, or Yin foods. Therefore, the mucilage is not just an optional nutrition but an essential, must-have nutrition if we want to live free from diseases and pain. And that's the point I want to get through.

The way the nature protects us appears to be very simple but is very effective as follows:

- Mucilage is normally taken in the meals of traditional foods in the forms of stone ground grains, roughages and variety of fruits, seeds and vegetables. Once again, mucilage is something slippery and sticky, or visco-elastic substances of our vegetarian foods.

- Some of the mucilage we eat is captured by the esophagus and stays on the walls of esophagus, and when water is drunk it washes down the esophagus and gets mixed in with the mucilage. This step is essential for proper hydration to take place, and without this step accomplished first no proper hydration occurs, no matter how much water one may drink. Period. So be serious about eating some mucilage rich foods most every meal and make it your lifetime habit. This can be your lifetime self-health insurance – by Mother Nature's bounty.

- Proper hydration is essential precondition for the nature's protection of our health and immunity to be built in. I believe the failure of proper hydration is potentially the underlying cause of all chronic diseases whatsoever and the recent sharp upticks in the incidence of several diseases such as follows: 1)

Type 2 diabetes, 2) So called degenerative diseases, 3) Dementia, 4) Digestive tract and Lungs and respiratory tract related epithelial tissue cancers, such as breast cancer, and especially those deadly cancers of pancreas and uterus, 5) Male as well as female infertility, 6) Premature births and related gestational anomalies. I can't possibly name all of them in this limited space, but it should suffice to say that since the nature's protection comes via nutrition and proper hydration the whole body is protected systemically as long as you eat from a reasonably proper diet, maintain your daily exercises, and stay enthused about your life.

- I see mucilage as the consort or an essential as well as an indispensable partner of water in our body. This mucilage/water partnership in our body is the cornerstone of human existence on earth, its resilience and survival through the eons to this day. It protected our health all along. This ancient truth has yet to be recognized and sink in the hearts of people especially those living in the modernized and developed world of ours today. There has been little consumer self-help natural health care education in this country. As a result people are completely left in the dark. Today's urban populations have long lost any cultural connection to their ancestral traditions in foods and self-care. Many experience serious health issues and run in and out of bankruptcies. Most major cities in America struggle with exploding homeless populations. Most people today seem to mistakenly believe that their health can be protected only via access to medical treatment and some kind of government program that would make the access available to average Americans with limited income. This has been a divisive issue in the U.S. and many other likewise industrialized countries of the world. There is deceptively an easy solution of this dilemma that bedevils our societies: just go out and teach them how to self-care by nutrition. It may take 5 to 10 years of lead time before the nature's protection should be fully implemented if everyone start taking my suggested nutrition today and continue to do so every day throughout your whole lifetime. The cost will be minimal to most everybody: a fraction of a dollar, or just a few dollars per day for a family, at the most on mucilage rich foods depending on what kind of foods you may choose.

- Since the invention of milling machines in the 1890's, however, some of us living in especially so called developed societies, choose to prefer denuded grains, which leave little mucilage to nourish and strengthen our bodies. As the result many of us suffer literally from various diseases!

- Think about that. We the people must muster our good senses and choose the correct path of this age old, natural proper self-care and never allow us to get distracted by the alluring barrage of quick fixes.

- Mucilage/water partnership is the cornerstone of our health and our existence on earth and we must build the edifice of our enjoyable life on earth and health on this cornerstone. And the strong constitution of our bodies can be founded only on this cornerstone with the following functional branches: 1) Lungs, respiratory channel and sensory organs, all smoothed by mucilage-turned-mucus, which directly communicate with nature, are all run smoothly trouble-free largely by epithelial cells as trained and provided for ages by nature; 2) The 27 feet long digestive tract, which communicates directly with nature at its both ends, from mouth to anus with its associated organs digests food and water and excretes the wastes and various toxins all well wrapped up tightly in mucilage-turned-mucus smoothly and trouble-free largely by epithelial cells, leaving the body harmless and ready for tomorrow, as trained and provided for ages by nature; 3) Reproductive-sexual-urinary system, using mucilage-turned-mucus, running the multiple differing functions smoothly trouble-free, successfully impregnates rarely troubled by so called "infertility", gestates the fetus for 10 lunar months trouble-free, and delivers on full term the next generation infant out into the bosom of Mother Nature and into the loving arms of its mother and father, to be suckled for a year or two and then raised to maturity—all these been done successfully for ages by our bodies' proper organs in direct communication with nature *NATURALLY!!!* Consider this to be the nature's ages old biotechnology, or simply the secrets of life.

Experiencing Dramatic Changes in Health

As I reflect on my own personal health issues and the inflammatory pressures I feel while getting old, I begin to suspect there may be more than what the eyes meet in the values and the roles of these interfacing structures toward our health, and I intend to look further into them in another chapter of its own. I see the potential of a far-reaching systemic protection of the wellbeing of an individual may be accorded by the interface, and by its as yet undefined extension of it.

The skin of my body has been ravaged by what I call inflammatory pressures, for the last nearly 5 years, itching all over making me go crazy, and still on-going for some time and eventually leaving me completely in peace in about 8 years since I started my mucilage rich food experiment. Before this itching episode started I was staying in Korea a few years to care for Mother until my brother and sister-in-law decided to take her back. Around that time I was experimenting with mucilage rich herbs such as what Americans know as Chinese yam, and called 'ma' in Korean. I also used leaves of molokheia grown in a corner of my yard, known to Americans as Egyptian spinach, and soaked seeds of flax and chia, using them interchangeably. During my last winter in Korea, 2013-14, I was given access to a few persimmon trees. They were young but tall trees standing on steep hills, bearing small fruit, known as pickling persimmons. They had little market value for the owner, but for me, a welcome bonanza. The fruit left on the trees into December and January, they turned soft and sweet. I loved to eat them and also enjoyed the idea of foraging for food. I cut a long bamboo pole for free and had fun with it. That was felt like a short-lived Shangri-la, but I forgot all about them long after when I left.

The direct link to itching has become gradually apparent over time for me to see, that was, my using mucilage rich foods. Early on while I was eating persimmons, though, I didn't experience any itching. When itching started I did have a reason not to quit eating them in spite of the itching, which was very aggravating indeed. Because also apparent to me were several huge health benefits that occurred at the same time and opened my eyes wide. My stool became well formed, firm, and delivered usually early morning regularly. That might have been expected in association with fiber. I used to be a shallow sleeper, often staying up into the small hours. But I started to sleep deep and thoroughly restful, often in long stretches 5 to 7 hours. I heard about people with insomnia and their relying on sleeping pills. I knew I was hitting big. But the thing most flabbergasted me was I found my leg muscles developed, and my thighs fattened out practically overnight. Unbelievable! I had been hiking aggressively for over the last 25 years every weekend, but strangely enough I never saw my leg muscles developed like my fellow hikers. I was one of the most aggressive and enthusiastic hikers in our group, but my thighs were thin and the lower legs were without the usual bulges. I didn't understand it. But I said to myself to explain that I had a condition called Yin Deficiency as they say in the Eastern Medicine, with the root of it probably in my childhood malnutrition, which is known to cause lifetime emaciation.

Encouraged by dramatic changes I have experienced since introduction of mucilage food into my diet I abandoned the earlier cautious approach and began adding up more mucilage to my food; which in turn made me drink more and more water to relieve itching. But eventually, I realized I couldn't go on like this any further and needed some help.

I went to see a doctor in spring 2015 after 40 years of abstaining from doing so. My doctor was a considerate and likable guy, and I trusted him. He told me my blood was so thin that I could have passed out, and sodium was so low that my kidney could have been damaged. But he said I was checked out fine. After giving me a week's regimen of prednisone and antibiotics, he sent me on to an ENT, who recommended both my eardrums to be punctured to help drainage, which was designed to keep infection in the area under control, and which in turn would help me hear better. I accepted it on the left but declined on the right because I felt it was good enough. Two months later I went back to my general practitioner, not the ENT, and asked him if he thought it appropriate to give me another round of antibiotics with prednisone. He agreed. And everything went so very well. The only difference, this time, from 40 years ago was in my diet, the mucilage food. There is not a shred of doubt in my mind. For 40 years I was completely shut out of the sense of smell and had hard of hearing more or less all along. Now at age 75, and first time in my adult life, my senses are brought up on tip-top condition. I now compare different types of cucumbers on the differences of their fragrances and enjoy as desert a half of small banana and prefer when it's fully ripe and full of dark spots on the skin with its enticing wonderful fragrances. I now enjoy listening to music at the minimum level of volume. Such changes have made me feel I'm no longer a dumb and insensitive person that I was, but my life is made worthy of living now.

I am not finished fighting itching, yet. Although the pressure is much less now it's still bothersome. By the time I finish writing the next chapter, I hope, I may find out a way to free myself from itching for good. And I'm working on it. (2/1/16) I have become completely free of any itching sometime after what I call the memorable event in May 2018. Complete details in Chapter Five.

Another thing I'm fighting now is the bloatedness of my stomach and its bulging. I have worn size 32 belt all my adult life. In the earlier years when I was hiking regularly, I remember I had my pants often slipping down a little and so had to be pulled up frequently. It was a bit annoying at the time. Now I have an opposite problem that is more than just annoying. My belt is so tight at its first hole that I often have to suck in to buckle myself. (Despite of this tightness I still resist extending to the next holes.) Last few months I have been trying to eat less on the one side, but I'm also cautious not to harm my constitution by a sudden jolt in my food intake. Last night I felt the itching pressure was much less but the dry mouth was somewhat worse, and made me quit drinking teas today. Upon waking up this morning, I ran my hand over my stomach and felt as if it got softened. How real this is or not, I don't know. I'll just keep doing my small step approach and see what happens. (2/13/16) I am still maintaining the same belt and its first hole. (9/17/18)

After stopping tea drinking I looked for some kind of broth to moisten my throat and mouth in the night, and tried juemingzi one day and night. The next day I tried wuweizi and gouqizi, 1 Tbsp each. The next day I used 2 Tbsp gouqizi, and 1 Tbsp wuweizi, and I liked it. (2/21/16)

Everything depends on water maintenance and control in intimate coordination with biorhythms such as heartbeat and breathing and in appropriate response to changes in the environment, and ultimately it boils down to such a delicate moment to moment open or shut down of all individual skin pores management is the intricate art of life keeping exercise. Consider the crudeness, insensibility, and stupidity of a supposedly intelligent and sensitive man totally neglecting his attention to the basic supplies, for years! I realize the gravity of my negligence. Now the challenge is how to get the natural biorhythm spontaneity restored to the skin pores. I have to learn the ways to live in tandem to those natural rhythms, but without trying to apply my artificial intelligence. Teach the old dog a new trick! But I have to give it a try. Mimic it. (2/22/16)

I feel so very good and deeply relaxed. I'm pretty sure now that I have reached where I have been aspiring to reach so frustratingly for so long – at least recent 5-6 years – especially in the last several weeks, making me feel within the final grasp of my goal. Last night I went to bed around quarter to 12 midnight, after drinking about 12 oz. of my brew in a 14 oz. mug. This was a lot of liquid just before going to bed, but I was led to believe that this might be the right amount I needed. I was awakened for urination perhaps around 4 a.m. judging from the light outside, and at the 2nd time it was 6:48, I felt so relaxed and well rested, so I got up for good. Today is market day and I want to start early, so I got to go now, and will return later. (3/09/16) Continued: What made me feel so good? Two things come to my mind.

One was that I stopped miso in my food, perhaps a lot of salt in it, which apparently contributed a great deal to my dry mouth. The other was I added 1Tbsp coconut flour to my brew last night. It consisted of 1) 2 Tbsp gouqizi, 2) 2Tbsp nuzhenzi, and 3) 1Tbsp wuweizi for about 10 days, and for the last 5 days I added to it 1 tsp raw cacao nibs

I got up 7:11 after my 2nd most deeply relaxing and peaceful night with no dryness of mouth whatsoever experienced and just one interruption for the need to urinate. If this can be repeated indefinitely night after night into the future, it suggests my body's water regulation has been fully restored. (3/10/16)

My brew has been quite sour with 1 Tbsp wuweizi, and I was concerned about it. Last night it hit me. I went to bed late at 1:08, got up 3:35, bit too early than expected, drank 12 oz of my brew, went back to bed, but got up again unexpectedly at 4:45. I found my skin hypersensitive and unbearably itching, which was contrary to recent trends. But the quality of itching was shallow like just on the very surface of it. I guessed it might be because my drink was too acidic, and after drinking 3-4 oz plain water, went back to bed. I got up for good 7:21, deeply relaxed as used to be but with a fairly strong dry mouth. Now I'm about to reduce wuweizi down to 1 tsp per day. (3/11/16)

I stopped using cacao nibs and coconut flour because I was having migraine headache before. This may be caused by protein imbalance. Once before I had this experience, I had stopped them and increased lysine rich protein sources like chicken, pork, tofu and beans. Then headache had soon disappeared. But not at this time! It lasted over a week. To fight it, I used 1 Tbsp coconut oil. It helped somewhat but not completely, so I took a tsp nutritional yeast last night. Although I do not know if it was responsible, but it's substantially gone. Maybe I should take some more of the nutritional yeast tonight. And I did immediately at 4 pm. (3/17/16)

I am now fully free of any itching and bloatedness is gone, too. (3/31/16) I used to blame the mucilage rich foods for all my itching, but I realize now that I am finally in a phase that I feel free from itching even though I continue consuming measured but steady amount of mucilage rich foods. I kept wondering if I could ever be free from itching while I would be still taking the same amount of mucilage rich foods. I figure that after several months passed since what I called the "memorable event" now I feel I am freed from being itchy. I intend to clarify this itchiness issue in an appropriate place in Chapter Five.

I have a reason to believe everything has gone well as I envisioned, and I found a way to live healthy ever after according to my proposition to have my daily food plan as my lifelong health plan. I dropped my brew with wuweizi, gouqizi, nuzhenzi, entirely, and in its stead I started making a clear what I call 'sea breeze soup' with a fresh in shell oyster, 2 prawns, 3 shell fish, an ounce piece of sockeye salmon, 2 small sweet potatoes, a half of golden beet root, 6 lianzi (lotus seeds), presoaked piece of kelp (about 2x4 inches dry), and 2 quarter inch slices of Chinese yam in two cups of water, and cooked for half an hour. The last 2 items were the strategic ingredients. The resulting soup worked beautifully for my purposes and was delicious and fulfilling as a meal as well. And there's just one minor incidental question: do I continue to need my nasal spray, or has it become toxic? I relied on it, and it made my life livable in the last 10 months. Now I have this question. I guess I need just a little more time to see how it's going to turn out. I am going now without using the spray. I had to use the 6 lotus seeds at supper as well. (4/2/16) So far so good! (4/3/16)

Dear Daughter:
I am writing about a bit of personal history on the very moments as they are very happening to share them with you.

I am sure you will be surprised and incredulous to hear about this: but I am sure now that I have outlasted the usefulness of my nasal spray you bought for me so long. It was expensive. But you didn't mind, when I said felt like needed it, and bought them for nearly 12 months. Now I'm sure I don't need it anymore, because my body won't tolerate it anymore. It would send me violent sneezes the kind I never experienced before. I felt couldn't risk them anymore so I abided a few days to see how it's going to turn out. I think I am tolerably doing well now on my own supposedly renewed natural mucus lining system alone, so I'm letting you know.

And thank you very much for all the supports you have so generously provided for so long and continuing. Thanks a lot, again.

Love,

Grateful Dad
(4/4/16)
(I sent an exact copy to my daughter in an email. It's a dream come true for me, at lo-o-o-ng last. It goes back to 1970's and at least 40 years.)

(I just used an ear wax remover, which I had long resisted, and removed a small piece of wax. I had poked my pinky repeatedly. Sometimes it helped.

This time the pinky alone didn't help. The little wax remover with 3 overlapping little circular scoops can be safely used and often with satisfying result.)

(That reminds me of my two little friends: my beloved traditional bamboo back-scratcher and a newfangled scratchy bath-towel scratcher. They were my godsend kept always close to me. They were serving night and day with soothing effect. I probably outlived their usefulness as well, but I'll still keep them around. They are dear to my senses.)
(4/4/16)

Alas! My rash decision to do away with my medical nasal spray all of a sudden abruptly threw me in the ditch of pain and misery in the eyes for days. I ordered some herbs to address those issues, while I don't even know if the herbs would lift me from these aggravations, I still have to wait for a week to arrive from Los Angeles. During the last 4-5 days I had to try to wash out my eyes of the offending substances by dropping 3 drops of almond oil into each of my eyes, about a dozen times altogether, and on recent couple of night, twice during the nights. I felt the draining from my left eye on 3 separate occasions, and then this morning I felt sort of a major draining from my right eye very first time, after which I felt the itching pressures in the eyes was noticeably lessened and made me feel somewhat relaxed. After which I immediately decided to wash my eyes out again. After I've done so with 3 drops of almond oil in each eye, I have become tolerably comfortable up until now. My right nostril is slightly starts itching. I think I'll repeat my almond oil in the eyes and through the nose. 1:45 pm, 4/8/16. I think I had verified the anti-inflammatory effect of my cacao nibs and coconut flesh tea in lessening my discomforts in the eyes. I have had trouble with amino acid imbalance troubles, which made me quit cacao-coconut tea for some time. Now that I strengthened the protein balance I'm going to regularize cacao-coconut intake either in soup or as a tea. In a single serving soup, my doze is 1/2 tsp nibs and 1 Tbsp coconut flakes. For an all day through night tea, I use 1 tsp nibs and 1 coffee spoonful, which is 2 Tbsp of coconut flakes, brought to boiled and simmered in 6 and 1/2 cups of water for 1/2 to 1 full hour. After drinking a 12 oz glass twice during the day after each meal I filled up that water and cooked again twice, so that I'll have refilled full 6 and 1/2 cups for the evening and through the night. 4/8/16

Last night I got up at 3:54, had so aggravated by the discomforts in the eyes, and couldn't go back to sleep. I had to do something. I dug through what I had in herbs and found two: pugongying root and tufuling root, and combined 12 g each, and boiled a tea. I brought it to a boil, then reduced heat setting to medium with lid slightly open, had it in a sustained boiling for 30 minutes, further reduced the heat setting to 9 o'clock position, watched for a while to make sure that it will continuously simmer at that level, and then I came down to my room, sat at my seat, fell overcome by sleep soon, waking up about 2 hours later at around 7:40. My eyes were painfully sensitive, watery and gummy and unable to keep them open. These were aggravations I had to go through because I was unwilling to use the medicated nasal spray called Nasonex, to see if I could come up with a reasonably comfortable procedure with my herbal medicine. Curiously, I was never focused on this. I have been focused during the last 3 years or so by using dietary regime that I considered to be the simple natural requirement, the Yin Food, or the Mucilage Food. Now that I am probably no sooner than barely restored in my Yin System than I had to deal with the resurgent my preexisting condition of sinusitis I realize was caught utterly unprepared. Well I should have been aware of it. Now I am prepared to tackle with it. I ordered appropriate herbs to address my sinus problems. In the mean time I have to smart myself from day to day until I'll get my supply in a few days. I am looking forward to the challenge. Now I think I'm prepared to successfully master this chronic illness one final time. At this juncture, I want to make a note that now I've got my mind back. It has been my constant concern that I must be losing my mind, and someday I may lose my mind totally and may be sent to an institution. But I feel like at this point as if my erstwhile forgetfulness is gone. I have to wait and see if it's true or not. Earlier this morning when I awakened prematurely, I felt strongly that way and said, "Now I've got my mind back!" (4/15/16)

I bought several herbs I thought essential and others I fancied wanted to try. None of the latter worked and was set aside. Cangerzi, shinyi, baizhi with my substituted bajito mint seems to be working. Initially I had difficulties and confusion due to excessive drying and infection in the nose. I cut back herbs in half from 6 g each down to 3 g each. Besides, I added 6 gram each of tufuling and pugongying to provide further cooling action. I'm considering adding still more: like machixian, and am curious about guizhencao, too. I also want to try adding shicangpu to see if it is helpful in managing polyps. A few weeks ago my daughter took me to the ENT, who noted large polyps in my nose, and I want to make sure they shall shrink away with my current herb formula, and if not, hopefully with the addition of shicangpu. My daughter demanded me to agree to go back to an ENT 6 months after moving to California, and made sure that the polyps are gone, or otherwise I must submit to the ENT procedure. I hope these will be the last steps wrapping up my long running self-healing by food endeavor successfully, although having to delve a bit into the professional herbal medicine was not initially envisioned. I had imagined that if I had eaten the

Yin Food enough it would restore my proposed The Yin System, which will help keep body free from most diseases if not all. But lately I had to concede the preponderant weight of a pre-existing condition wasn't washed away. And my own need to be restored in health tops everything else. At this time, my Yin has been largely restored but there is still a big step short. I know this because my current herbal formula would work for me only when I eat 2 dried persimmons a day, one each cooked in my morn and evening meals. Having taken the herbs caused my eyes constantly wet and unbearably itchy, and or my nostrils extremely itch and there was no peace. But with persimmons eaten everything is calmed down, becomes normal and in peace. There is no nasal congestion whatsoever. I just have to keep myself warm, and eat warm food only. I have just decided and I will eat or drink nothing direct from the refrigerator again. I had a real bad experience today after eating lunch out of the refrigerator. Not again! I just have had a hot cup of my herbal tea. It makes me feel good. I think it is pretty good and working nicely. I don't feel there is any kind of obstruction in my nose. But I would like to hear an ENT declare he finds no polyps in my nose. It is my hope that all of the above will be accomplished after moving to California, which is scheduled for the 8th of June. (5/14/16)

Yesterday, 5/31/16, My daughter took me with her two kids to view Lincoln Memorial in Washington, DC. Something was in my mind when I woke up 4 am. I tried to fall back to sleep but I couldn't. Too much excitement! Finally, at 5:17 I got out of the bed, got dressed, and, with an umbrella in my hand just in case, went out on a walk in the early morning dusk before sunrise. While walking, my mind has been busy making changes in my life, from a sluggish senior on his sunset mind into a seasoned old Eastern medicine professional returned to practice, realizing my dream of being a good doctor, keeping my patients in good health. My Important foods include, but not limited to, persimmon, almond/coconut milk, and the little lotus seeds. I imagine or practically may be engineering my rejuvenation and pushing myself out of the long doldrums. I begin to think this is truly happening to me now. From a late evening morose lazy old owl of a man may be changing back to my early rising, energetically and consciously uplifting old self and begin to renew my old hope of working up to my 100th year and make it into a plan that will be actually implemented step by step. The plan may get started once I moved to California, which is to come a week from today. (6/1/16)

Although I had often talked about rejuvenation in the past I have been rather dismissive of real rejuvenation lately. But I begin to feel a subtle change occurring in my body. I used to feel my upper body was heavy and stiff, tended to fall forward, and to resist it and stand upright was hard and cumbersome. Now it seems the weight I used to feel is quite lightened, the stiffness is probably not there anymore. If I continue walking the trails as I have since having arrived here the 8th of June. I was long wondering about those fellow hikers in their late 70's and into the 80's who were walking the trails better than, and often ahead of some of the younger ones in the group, and why I will never be like them. Now I begin to feel differently and hopeful. I'll continue to walk the trails and once or twice a week I'll go up on the mountain trails whatever they may turn out to be. My son Eric called me today to say Happy Father's Day to me with all of his children, one after another. (6/20/16) I visited his family around the Fourth of July, and had fun hiking with all the children for 5 hours. It took long because I was slow but I enjoyed it very much and had another short and easy hike after resting a day.

I am still walking one and half to two hours every day in the cool of the early morning. My body feels lighter and less burdensome as I continue walking. I intend to keep it up as long as I can. And my current diet helps maintain trouble free nasal cavities and makes me feel great. I must stay keen on protein balance, that is, lysine over arginine. I add a spoon of almond flour to my food, and use a drink or two of almond/coconut milk with mulberry juice in the night. For protein I use a small slice of salmon (morning), an egg (lunch), a small slice of skirt steak (evening), and often add some tofu and or home cooked dry beans and or lentils. Besides, I have to balance out the drinks of almond/coconut milk by goat milk yogurt or cheese. Among my staple of vegetables are: seaweed, green beans, golden beetroot, broccoli with stems, turnips, radishes, sweet potatoes, kabocha squash, celery, asparagus, etc., and some herbs. (7/24/16)

Soon after moving back to California in June 2016, I replaced almond/coconut milk and mulberry juice and instead chose pomegranate juice and the unsweetened the Original Almond Milk as the beginning of my permanent dietary solution of my chronic sinus problem without using any medication whatsoever. I believe that this combination worked very well with my continuing background treatment of mucilage rich foods. Complete details will be given in the final chapter, which I plan to make the epitome of my self-care regimen. About 4 years later, now on April 27, 2020, I feel assured that all my residual morbidities have been completely wiped out, and that my use of juices of mulberries and pomegranates, the two fruits I thought to be the most enriched in Yin, were certainly helpful in minimizing my discomforts, and the almond/coconut milk may have been instrumental in circumventing my body's allergic tendencies. All in all, the ultimate foundation of healing of my body was certainly

based on my very own purposefully adopted habit of consuming plenty of fiber rich or mucilage rich foods every day, and as a result of that habit, as I theorized, my esophagus must have been fully smeared by the "s*lippery and sticky stuff*", so that whenever I drank water it must wash down some of the "*slippery and sticky stuff*" and gets mixed up with it by the time it reaches the stomach. And this very process changes the very nature of water from a lifeless inorganic substance into an organic living person's body water. This is probably a piece of new information for you. However, this very process   accomplishes *HYDRATION/HYDRATION/HYDRATION.*   Without   this process allowed to happen first, regardless however much or how often you may drink water, the inorganic water is not allowed to enter your intimate realm of organic entity without first itself being changed organic. And that's why my disease got continuously worse and worse for nearly 50 (yes, fifty) years, but it reversed the course back 8 years ago, when I started my food only experiment *With NO MEDICATION WHATSOVER,* gradually but unmistakably proceeded toward the full recovery, of which I here and now ascertain this Monday, April 27, 2020. I proved through my personal pain in my own personal body and learned that just drinking water does not accomplish hydration. So don't say that or repeat that to me. I know it's a lie. If you still say that, you are a liar. Liar, liar, your pants on fire!

I have been here fully two months in Los Gatos, California. I took advantage of the Los Gatos Creek Trail walking about two hours every day since I arrived here on the 8th of June, 2016. At first it was very difficult because I felt as if my upper body was too heavy and might fall flat on the ground. I wondered how some of my erstwhile hiking buddies in the Angeles Mountains seemed to be walking well and wondered what was wrong with me. Now I realize it was because I practically stopped walking in the last 15-20 years, which is not really true. If I had access to trails I should have continued walking. The sickly heaviness of the upper body gradually lifted over the last two months, with the heaviness sensation slowly being lowered to the buttocks, and then lastly to the knees albeit briefly. Now I am free from that sickly heaviness, but I am not back to the younger person that I was. I am still an old person getting older every day. But I expect, in the weeks and months ahead, that I may carry myself somewhat more lightly, if not energetically. It remains to be seen. (8/08/16)

Chapter 4

HOW THE YIN SYSTEM GUARDS THE HEALTH

My First Experiences with Mucilage Rich Foods
When I consider the epithelial cells as exterior communication agents with nature, some ancient health lore seemed to make sense. I knew about slippery elm (Ulmus rubra syn. U. fulva) lore of the Native American peoples and the early pioneers of the North American Continent from reading a book on the pioneers' life. Later in 1995, when I was enrolled in Samra University of Oriental Medicine, I got attracted by an ad offering a weeklong seminar by a noted botanist and author at an herb farm of Chinese medicine located in the state of Missouri in that summer.

And later I learned of okra gumbo dish of early French immigrants known as Creole people in what eventually became Louisiana later, which became a famous southern dish and later served at Senate in Washington; and what was known as sarsaparilla among early Hispanic settlers of Middle America in what is now known as Venezuela and the neighboring countries, which was reputed as effective on syphilis; and another lore of an Egyptian pharaoh of North Africa, getting healed of his chronic illness by eating the leaves of jute plant in his soup, and the plant is known as Molokheia in Egyptian, or Egyptian spinach, or Jew's jute plant to some Americans.

In the Far East, Chinese, Korean and Japanese peoples cooked tubers of what is known to Americans as Chinese yam or cinnamon vine root (tuber) and other herbs in similar ways. In all of these differing regions around the globe they used the herbs with highly touted health claims, which were widely respected by the local peoples.

Some of these herbs may still have large following in their local areas. Molokheia is said to be one of the most popular vegetables in today's Egypt and several neighboring countries in the Middle East. Knowing what I know, this is quite understandable, and it is good for the people. The Chinese yam, known as 'ma' in Korea, has small number of definitely very loyal clientele that buys the tuber year after year. But few people outside the areas paid any attention on the healing potential of these herbs. They are practically buried in the local mouth to mouth folklore and are largely ignored.

And I also came to get familiarized with flax seeds from the Middle Eastern region, and chia seeds from Mexico and Central America. These seeds when soaked in water produce thick gel like the other herbs I mentioned above. These qualities were recognized and highly valued by the local people for their perceived health benefits.

I started studying these herbs and began to use them in my diet in various ways. As I did, I realized that all these plants shared a common characteristic among them that they were all rich sources of mucilage, or soluble fiber.

Epithelial Cells as Yin Front Lines

But the outline of them has already become clear to me. Most of them had various health claims of either stopping diarrhea or constipation, or helping digestion, or sometimes asthma, cough or breathing, or urinary system related complaints, etc. I was able to perceive immediately that all of the complaints are somehow related to the organs that are serviced by epithelial tissues such as, digestive organs, respiratory organs, and Kidney/reproductive/urinary organs. The various health claims made by the lore all reported either of the lung troubles or digestive troubles, or the reproductive and urinary organ related troubles. This was one of the first hints directing my search.

Epithelial cells work as body's customs agents in all imports and exports of resources and wastes. Everything that enters or leaves body must clear through epithelial cells. They are the body's primary agents in receiving, processing, and distributing the food, water, and air; and take care of their waste products so they will be properly readied to be excreted on timely basis; and serve all the sense organs, eyes, ears, tongue and skin.

First Hint: The Ancient Lore Made Sense

I have associated that problem with mucous membrane system and somehow got a hint of it may be related to mucilage after I bought and ate some long tubers of Chinese yam, also known as cinnamon vine or 'ma' in Korean. As I liked ma I did some research and came to know the mucilage was a water soluble kind of fiber and there were other rich sources of similar soluble fiber, and that I already had some in my possession, namely, chia seeds and flax seeds. This was a huge break that ushered me into what I thought my desperately searched solution territory. The mucilage contained in those plant tissues seemed to be consistent with the ancient folklore. The improvements that seem to be happening in my body like my nose and my guts seemed to belong to each of the respiratory and digestive systems to correspond to the details of the folklore, although I wasn't sure to which department my deep sleep improvement should belong to. And so I started using them. To draw mucilage I soaked them in small amount of water for a few hours and then I tried to chew the swollen seeds. Somehow, I sensed that the liquid mucilage released from the seeds was the main product that I was seeking. But there was no easy way to separate the liquid from the seeds, and apparently the seeds are likely to hold more mucilage that may be released later. And so I chose to swallow the whole thing, water and the seeds, in my salad or soup. It was obviously a little accommodation I needed to make but for me expecting huge health benefits to gain from eating them potentially it was not at all a difficult one.

A few years ago, from January 2010 to August 2014, when I stayed in Korea I planted molokeia, an herb known from the famous Egyptian lore in my garden. I found its mucilage was very slippery, and arguably even more so than flax seeds and ma. And since my encounter with the herb was the first one, I was cautious of using molokeia. But now with experience of different textures of mucilage, I came to prefer the most slippery one because of my impression of it flushing out the nasal mucus more easily and better. But my plants I planted this year in my Virginia garden didn't do so well to provide me the herb. I had thought that herb was easy to grow but I am disappointed. Next year I must do better. The most herbs I'm using this year have been mostly frozen okra bought in the stores, next flax seeds, last was occasional ma. Because farmers in Virginia and the neighboring southern states grow okra as one of the popular regional specialty vegetables, it was the cheapest and the easiest thing to obtain any time around the year, and I tended to use it the most. They come both fresh and frozen and are available the year around, but only known to some. You may have to look for them.

That was probably when I first experienced a profoundly deep sleep "like a baby" and I immediately associated it with ma and soaked flax seed usage. And since then, this deep sleep was practically reenacted most every time I slept. This was quite unexpected and pleasantly surprised me. Much through my adult life years I was a late and shallow sleeper, often interrupted or had difficulty of falling back to sleep. Because I wasn't often sleepy in the night, I used to stay up very late, often 12 or 1 and sometimes to 2 or 3. And I used to think that my unsatisfactory sleeping habits are due to my Yin Deficiency or chronic dehydration, and that the deep sleep I experienced in many recent months was probably owing to the recent use of okra, flax seeds and occasional ma.

Now I want you to recall each of all the herbs I talked about in the beginning produces copious mucilage that is slippery to your fingers as well as to your mouth. This mucilage is very slippery because it contains water soluble fiber, or something called mucilage, which is one of the most essential nutrients, in my opinion, it is as much as essential as proteins, carbohydrates and fats all put together. Because our current science doesn't recognize its proper position in natural human health keeping it's still in the dark. This is the one nutrient that is largely missing in our current consciousness of our diet to a great detriment to our health. I view this nutrient as an antithesis to all the energy producing foods such as protein, fats, and carbohydrates in terms of fighting diseases, and as such diametrically essential to balanced human nutrition.

In my opinion, it regulates human health and prevents disease if it is allowed to participate, for this serves as Yin food in the grand scheme of things against its counterpart, the better-known trio set of essential nutrients: proteins, carbohydrates and fats, which collectively serve as Yang food. I believe this is true throughout the entire evolutionary process of human race just as it is today.

Because our current consciousness of nutrition sciences chiefly concentrate on those energy producing foods and largely neglect non-energy producing nutrients that would counter-balance it in the interest of health maintenance and disease control: The water with fiber dissolved in it, our society is prone to developing a host of diseases that would have been prevented if this naturally essential nutrition were in place and its proper balancing act were recognized. And most modern so called degenerative diseases that are ultimately caused by chronic dehydration, which is caused in turn by failure of proper hydration, which is caused by lack of this essential nutrition in the system. In other words, our diet is deficient of the natural nutrient that would have protected our bodies from disease and instead precariously skewed on the Yang side, which is Heat promoting by nature, without the antagonizing and therefore counter-balancing influence of its cooling Yin food. The Yin food is the one to give proper balance to our current diet far skewed on the Yang side. All

other talk of balance is gone to waste without having the balance of Yin food versus Yang food restored first, because it is the most vital one that truly matters in the broadest sense of physical health. If this is placed back in its proper context where it deserves to be, all of its ills will have a chance to be corrected, potentially. This is the law of nature, which was placed in our bodies from time immemorial. We have to understand this and embrace it wholeheartedly. This is the essence of my simple dream of realizing a disease-free society. What would be the monetary cost of realizing this largely disease-free society? I think the cost will be relatively minimal, something most of us can well afford, a fraction of a dollar or a dollar or two at the most per day.

The Constitution of a Physical Body

The Constitution of a physical body defined as presented earlier is understood to be "the physical makeup of the individual comprising inherited qualities modified by environment." The definition is a highly abstract linguistic expression, and it has its use. But when we talk about a living human body we need a lot more descriptive terms to convey what we mean to say. If I may repeat what I said earlier, this is a living body, a self-standing, -defending, -maintaining, –healing integral individual entity, that is free-roaming in nature. This body is not ever living or omnipotent. But the body has developed such an incredibly sophisticated self-perpetuating life-support system out of seemingly simple things found ubiquitous in nature that boggles my mind. It certainly demands my utmost respect, and as a token of my respect I want to capitalize the word Constitution. When I use the terms like "integral individual entity" to describe The Constitution I mean it to be integrating the one whole human body as a living entity, and at the same time it constitutes the bottom core of its physical existence. In other words, I mean the Constitution is to be the bottom core of what it makes to be a self life sustaining individual system. When life is conceptualized as being born of and sustained by continued opposition between the forces of Yin and Yang, a sort of a duel ending up as a comingling never ending seemingly friendly dance of the duo, I should characterize the Constitution as the Yin of the body. Therefore, when I call it the Yin of the body I mean it to be the same as "the bottom core of what it makes to be a self life sustaining individual system."

Inflammation and Inflammatory Pressures

The Yin of the body is under attack. Symbolically speaking, I could say, with some theatrical exaggeration, a fire is raging across the prairie of North American continent: the land mass that was once completely covered by tall grasses, and the fire being the inflammatory pressure building in the bodies of Americans, who refuse to eat 'grasses' saying "I'm not a rabbit," and would rather eat from cattle that was raised and fattened in a factory farm with corn, soybean, and antibiotics, and made readily available relatively cheap and around the clock by refrigeration. How long human beings have been able to look something under the microscope? Have we overlooked something that is in plain view and failed to connect the dots with the average smart with which we humans survived and prospered these hundreds and thousands of sheaves and sheaves of years? This sudden dietary change in the humanities is going to turn out O.K.. Because our consciousness is often shaped by our daily exposure in the surroundings where we live – shifting this way and that all the time. Although our individual lives are relatively short or long depending on how you view them and go through many changes like growing up, going to school, working, getting married, changing jobs, etc., etc., there is one constant thing we often tend to forget that you remain the same unique individual body born of your parents. In case you fail there is no replacement – end of the story. Therefore, consider your body as a vehicle your persona rides that is irreplaceable and priceless. But who cares about the upkeep of your vehicle, which is your body? Who is it that can secure and maintain The Constitution of your body strong throughout your life and down to your last day? It must be you, and no one else is responsible for it. Not the doctors, certainly, but you! You should take the personal charge of it and there is a world of difference if you do. This priceless machine needs to be maintained by daily intake of proper food and water day in and day out. Your food makes your body. Care should be taken, therefore, in choosing what to eat and drink, for a proper maintenance practice would lead to trouble free running of your vehicle throughout your lifetime. In spite of any number of changes you may face in your life, as long as you stick with the basic diet that sustained the human species until today, I strongly reassure you that the odds are in your favor. Don't get distracted by the recent noise the proponents of medical care stirs up these days, for you are in good hands – in Mother Nature's perennial care.

The Well-being of Our Children and Grandchildren

I lost one of my three younger brothers to heart attack in his 60's and his son, my nephew, at the same fate in his 40's leaving a toddler boy an orphan. My father, a poor peasant farmer with a growing family, but with smart skills and enterprising spirit was cut short at his age 36 leaving my poor mother straddled with four young children including a newborn to be fed and clothed. My mother apparently felt *abandoned* by my father and never recovered from the shock. She never told us a word and kept a dead silence about our father. And he himself was left an orphan, having lost both his parents at a tender age 5 to a cholera epidemic in South Korea. I lost my maternal Grandmother, the only Grandmother I ever met and loved, in circumstances that still make me feel sorry. I once helped her cross the village river in a small boat. I should have been 7 or 8 years old at the most. When I crossed her and let her off safely on the other side she was pleased and proudly called me "A Son of a Boat." She later chose to come over to relieve her daughter, my mother, after my father had an operation to relive of his swollen abdomen and later, he checked into a clinic to recover from the surgery, my Grandmother volunteered to come and stay with my father at the clinic looking after him. There was a taboo against a mother-in-law to come over for her son-in-law's illness, nonetheless. One day my mother must have sent me over to check on my father and Grandmother. While visiting there I became aware of certain noise, shot out of the door, and witnessed my Grandmother suddenly collapsing with some frothy saliva spilling out of a corner of her mouth and apparently soon thereafter passed away. I don't remember who told me to run. But I ran all the way home – a perhaps well over a 5K, alerted my mother and then ran out again another 5K or two and alerted my uncles. These two young men, my middle uncle about 17 or 18 years of age at the time, and the eldest uncle in his early 20's, suddenly informed of having lost their mother out of the blue, had to walk the distance of several 5K runs with a make-shift bamboo carrier, picked up their mother's lifeless body and had to walk all the way back home, how utterly devastated they should have been!!!

And in a few months thereafter it so happened during the Korean War my eldest uncle was taken captive while working in his rice field by the invading North Korean Army. While being forced to march with the Communists my uncle got shot on his lower leg and was left behind when they retreated in haste. It so happened that a passerby farmer who happened to know my parents took notice that the injured young man left alone on the roadside looked alike my mother and he started a conversation with my uncle. That's how the neighbor man brought my injured uncle on his back carrier to my mother in the middle of the night. Oh, how grateful we all felt to the kindly neighbor! My uncle is safe now and is in the care of my mother. I watched my mother with a fascinated boyish admiration how expertly she went about treating my uncle's gunshot wound. First of all, she brought out a couple of dark blankets and draped them over the front entrance and back window. This was a precautionary measure not to attract any attention by the air surveillance during the war. It became a way of living at the time. My mother, an uneducated country woman obviously hasn't had any experience or any supplies either or anything related to medical stuff but seemed to be proceeding with calm confidence. She brought in her own supplies ready: a clean washing bowl with fresh water, a few spoonfuls of well fermented homemade miso and a few slabs of freshly made tofu, which she made earlier in the day in preparation for the approaching Fall Festival or Chuseok. After washing out the wounds she spooned the miso directly on the raw flesh and placed the slices of tofu on top of it and then she wrapped the whole thing secure around my uncle's leg with strips of her own homemade white cotton cloth. That was it. It apparently worked beautifully. My uncle's gunshot wounds got healed completely without any complications. As luck would have it, when the gunshot went through his leg, there were no bones touched! A clean healing resulted! This little story may not seem to be directly related to my ongoing narratives of Mother Nature's protection of our heath and safe maintenance. But I thought it illustrated a snapshot that could have happened to anybody and it showed how we humans survived when we were struck by unusual circumstances. I would rather have a broad view of things and not get lost at the current tight circumstances. I would rather view the immense whole human evolutionary history and draw an effective lesson that may apply to my life today and beyond. And that's what I am trying to do in this little book.

My point is that much of these tragedies are preventable if we were aware and acted to prevent them from happening to us. I think I have discovered the simple natural protection of human health and survivability throughout the entire human evolutionary history on earth. I have identified that simple natural protective nutrient is something called *mucilage,* or soluble fiber dissolved in water solution. This has been ubiquitous on earth both on land or water. And I also said earlier that in the Traditional Eastern Medicine in the Orient a substance defined as Yin Essence was identical to mucilage. This nutrient is so essential to human health and survival including freedom from disease as well, and that a proper hydration cannot be accomplished without this nutrient. So I call it a necessary condition *sine qua non* for proper hydration to take place in human body. I believe this is how the Mother Nature's protection of human health and the unlimited survivability of human race ultimately work. Now I have adopted my daily consumption of mucilage rich foods as my personal healthcare program and I am inundated with calm inner happiness.

I feel like going on top of the hills and screaming: "Here's the way the Mother Nature takes care of us all! This is the true and permanent solution of personal healthcare!"

Admittedly, there is a substantial lead time required before one can see the full benefit and get a personal assurance thereof. And in my case, it took 6-7-8 years. And it is quite a bit of time. True! But I believe the process is worth waiting for. I believe this time is well spent by the body, rehydrating itself cell by cell, and thus removing the fake and replacing back the truly hydrated cells, and thus rooting out the disease completely. And this is how I see the time taking process. I hate to use a term so thoroughly maligned and deservedly so, but I am sure in my whole consciousness and declare "**It is truly a unique and the ultimate potential cure-all!!!**"

It is my understanding that this proposition is replicable personally to any person who is willing to use mucilage rich foods as described in this book twice a day and everyday continuously without stopping for several years, and if satisfied, continue to use the mucilage rich foods as a measure to protect your health throughout your life. And as a result, you will find that your health seems well protected and secure.

Any Side Effects or Discomforts for the Trial? Yes, there are some — pesky itching problem, which lasted for nearly 5-7 years in my case, then decreased somewhat and finally completely disappeared soon thereafter, and the in-sleep dry mouth problem. I was first startled to have in-sleep dry mouth, which made my mouth shut and dry one night 10 years ago about 2008. I got struck with great fear. At the time I had retained cans of herbal powders from my previous Glendale, CA clinic. So, I took one teaspoonful of dried plum powder and as soon as I put it in my mouth I was quickly flooded with rich saliva, which made me comfortable again. But the effect was short lived. Never again it would work. I renewed a widened search and 2 years later I moved back to Korea to take care of my aging mother and settled in a countryside home. The rest is the story I tell in this book. I believe that condition was just one of the symptoms of my body-wide chronic dehydration and has been cured for good by my recent use of mucilage rich foods, and therefore is no longer of concern. But I am still bothered a bit slightly by a different kind of dry mouth now. This current dry mouth is caused by my peculiar embarrassing recent habit. Let me explain: I have been using full dentures for more than three decades. Normally I would brush them with disinfectant toothpaste. But I found the task loathsome and often feel too lazy to do so. Occasionally, food scraps are left in and I wash them out with plain water. When I did that, I often get sore gum, which I see as inflamed possibly by sugary residues from eating dried apricot as desert. Now I eat my apricot desert not after the meal but chew it mixed with the meal and stopped brushing entirely. That may leave some food residues in my mouth but keeps it clean from any infection and no more sore gum stuff anymore! It's a bit awkward, though, to drop a lifelong habit of brushing teeth. As a result, I endure a bit of dry mouth around the end of the nighttime sleep. As soon as I wake up saliva flows quickly. I take the trade-off as fair enough. Now as of April 19, 2019 all those itching discomforts are completely gone. Thank you!

The Potential Benefits: Too Numerous to Name All

I will just present a short outline, but remember that I am talking with a sweeping view through the entire human evolutionary existence in my mind, and I present the same in a simplified formula as follows:

Your Mucilage Rich Foods Eaten Daily = Proper Hydration Accomplished
= Your Health Protection by Mother Nature Activated
=Free from All Organic Diseases and Free from Pain Due to Diseases

In my opinion, this formula offers the most effective, and the most comprehensive lifelong healthcare protection at the least expense possible to everybody, who is willing to eat the mucilage rich foods, because it is intimately built into the very biology of our bodies since the very beginning of human evolution on this earth. You just help the ages-old and wise body of yours do the natural thing it does best. With enough mucilage in your system, currently certain widespread health problems such as insomnia and erectile failure will be wiped out clean, which I know from my firsthand experience, and I would normally expect that many childbearing age women's various gynecological health issues eased off and more women may choose and opt for natural birth at home or with midwives and show less interest in Caesarean procedure. And I also expect that older women may not experience menopause at their usual age but likely to be delayed many years, or possibly never at all. I don't know if this potential situation would be a blessing or a curse, but I say it may be in the offing. And in this regard, I'd like to view the biblical story that Abraham's old wife Sarah bore him a child in her 100th year might have been possible naturally. But I am pretty sure that it is entirely possible that an older woman who has eaten the mucilage rich foods throughout her entire life may never experience the so-called vaginal dryness in her later life. Any copycat couples of Abraham and Sarah may be in the offing in the next 100 years if this dietary measure I advocate fans out widely.

Just keep in mind all the time that you are the ultimate decision maker on what to eat and what to drink. Keep the idea of balance in your mind all the time. And make sure that anything that may be toxic or hallucinogenic not to enter your body. That's all there's to it. I believe that this natural process was responsible for human race to have survived so far, and will keep protecting us throughout our lifetimes, and beyond likewise.

History Sometimes Can Be Full of Ironies like the one told by a scientist named Deanna Pucciarelli. According to her article that "delineates the historic trajectory of cocoa consumption, the linkage between cocoa's bioactive-mechanistic properties, paying special attention to nitric oxides role in vasodilation of the arteries, to the current indicators purporting the benefits of cocoa and cardio-vascular health", Alfred Nobel of Norway, a once chemistry student under a Russian teacher and in the road construction family business visited Paris to study under a famous chemistry teacher there, upon hearing that a new chemical nitric oxide (NO) caused an explosion. He brought the material back home and eventually invented gunpowder and the rest is history. While staying in Paris he experienced chest pain (angina pectoris) and his doctors recommended nitric oxide of all things. Cocoa has been used for chest pain since around year 1500, and its effective chemical was just been identified as nitric oxide and he was unable to make up his mind. According to the same article, Alfred Nobel "Seven weeks before his death he wrote:

My heart trouble will keep me here in Paris another few more days at least, until my doctors are in complete agreement about my immediate treatment. Isn't it the irony of a fate that I have been prescribed N/G 1 (nitroglycerine), to be taken internally! They call it Trinitrin, so as not to scare the chemist and the public.

He was apparently too much aware of its explosive power and let it pass. "It was not until the 1970," according to the article, "researchers returned to investigate the relationship between NG and vasodilation of the coronary arteries." The final one after a long list of ironies in the Alfred Nobel's relationship with N/G was enacted: "On October 12, 1998", when "1998 Nobel Prize in Physiology or Medicine was awarded … The Nobel Prize founded on the discovery of nitroglycerine 150 years earlier, which was used as a detonator to blow through granite and create tunnels was now recognized, in its related NO derivative, for playing a role in opening up biological tunnels (arteries)."

But her Real story is here: "Linkage between Cocoa and Heart Health The Kuna Indians live on San Blas islands off coast of Panama. A segment of the Kuna population had migrated to Panama City for economic opportunities and other reasons. Researchers recognized that the Island-Kuna had very low incidence of hypertension when aging, whereas the Mainland-Kuna hypertension levels were similar to other urban dwelling people. The hypertension increases with age and is considered a risk factor for cardiovascular disease (CVD). The island Kuna had little age-related hypertension and researchers looked at environmental factors, including diet, that might explain the difference. What they discovered was that Island

Kuna but not Mainland-Kuna, drank five cups of cocoa per day. Moreover, the type of cocoa the Island-Kuna consumed to be flavonoid-rich (900 mg/day) and the differences in low prevalence of hypertension were seen greatest in older rather than younger people. Other factors were investigated, such as differences in tobacco use, but were ruled out as contributory.

"The relationship between consumption of high levels of cocoa and cocoa containing products and low levels of hypertension also were found in another older population located thousands of miles away in Holland. This prospective study focused on older men (Zutphen Elderly Study) and data were collected 15 years post-baseline. A cross-sectional analysis measuring habitual cocoa-containing products was determined to be inversely associated with high blood pressure and prospectively related to cardiovascular mortality. The association between high levels of cocoa consumption and heart health outcomes gained international attention in the mid 1990s, and research to determine the nutrients inherent in cocoa that may play a role in this relationship began in earnest during this time.

"Flavonoids a subclass of polyphenols are abundant in fruits and vegetables and manifest in nature in many forms. The most commonly consumed and richest source of flavonoids in foods are quercetin and kampferol. Although generally low in concentration (--15 to 30 mg/kg) on a wet weight basis, these nutrients are found in onions, apples, and blueberries, products that are core foods in most American diets."

By Deanna L. Pucciarelli, **Cocoa and Heart Health: A Historical Review of the Science** at www.ncbi.nim.nih.gov PMC3820048

Flavonoids, richest source foods, and health benefits

Chapter 5

A SELF NURTURING WAY OF LIVING

Nurture your body for health. You are the only one to ensure it!
Nurture your spirit for happiness. You are the only one to guarantee it!

The Background Where I Come From
I was born and raised with three younger brothers in Korea, and lost my father when I was just 9 years old. We were dirt poor. Our mother struggled to feed and clothe us. As children all of us were malnourished. As a toddler I often had seizures and my mother had to run to the village doctor carrying me on her back. "Where are you going with your dead child?" People used to ask her, she told me.

And I often broke out in large hives, which I remember. She brushed me with mugwort tea. When I was older she told me to gather some mugwort that was growing under the hedges. She juiced it and gave me the bitter juice to drink. She told me it would strengthen my stomach and guts. I knew some kids crying and throwing a tantrum not to swallow a bitter medicine. But I was obedient like a "good child," and drank every bowl she gave me without complaining. I never talked back or rebelled to my mother. I was praised as an exemplar child by everybody in my neighborhood. I realized much later that my failure to articulate and assert myself against my mother's authority cost me dearly in my adult life. It was like a self-inflicted curse over the entire course of my life setting back my personality from its natural blossoming.

While growing up food was always scarce. "Pasting the mouths," as Koreans used to say, that is, feeding our selves, was a great challenge. My mother had to add wheat bran, an almost animal feed, to stretch her supplies of barley and chunks of it filled half of my lunch box taken to school.

At lunch time kids used to trade their side dishes called banchan in Korean but I was too embarrassed and kept to myself away from my classmates, which perhaps helped launch me to be a self occupied loner.

While serving in the Korean Army for a year and half, the compulsory service as a college student, they gave me a bowl of rice with a bowl of miso soup 3 times a day, 7 days a week. But I had diarrhea most every day. Looking back, I was weak and sickly as a young man. But I liked to think I was healthy. I hadn't had the least idea of how to care for myself. As I worked for 7 years as a newspaper reporter in Korea I was taken to heavy drinking to fit in the culture, which probably didn't help my health either.

In my early 30's I came to the U.S., studied advertising obtaining a master's degree at the University of Illinois at Urbana-Champaign, and moved to, lived in Chicago. My memory there was of bitterly cold winters. In a few years I got hay fever. An allergist said I had several allergies and allergic rhinitis. Looking back, it was the beginning of a chronic illness that tortured me for decades. I was racked by asthma attacks in the wee hours of the morning, piercing migraine day and night and debilitating lethargy all the time. My nasal cavities were swollen red and full of noxious dark purplish mucus. A stubborn infection blocked my airways completely and I couldn't breathe. How I endured all that, I wonder now, decades later.

My doctor gave me strong antibiotics for months but didn't help at all. I was referred to an ENT doctor and asked him if surgery might help. My wife pushed me for surgery. The doctor said it might not help but he was willing to do it if I wanted. Out of desperation I had to try it.

The next year she pushed me for another surgery. Completely exhausted bodily as well as spiritually, I couldn't but comply with her wishes. None of these surgeries, however, gave me even a moment of relief. Any food I ate seemed to aggravate it. A death seemed to be a real possibility.

I agreed to divorce and moved to Los Angeles with my one-year old baby girl. It was so painful to leave my 8-year old son behind with his mother and walk away. I adored him and loved him so very much. I wanted to keep both children with me. The day I packed my personal belongings and left him he cried convulsively jumping up and down, tearing my heart out. But I had to turn my back and walk away. I thought I would get him back somehow but it never turned out that way. I never saw him again until he knocked on my door one day at his age 19.

Now back to my story. I had hard time working and caring my baby alone. Eventually, I had my mother to come over from Korea, help me raise my little girl. But when I said no to her recommendation for Holy Ghost faith healers, my mother turned and cursed, as she blurted out, "You will never get well unless you go back to God."

She suggested then I try moxibustion. It was a device filled with mugwort connected to a manual air pump, which reminded something that looked like a giant smoking pipe. You lit the herb and squeeze the pump. It was placed on the nape of my neck, tied with a scarf to make it stay there. As I squeezed it the hot air burned into my flesh eventually making a hole. But I did it for half an hour everyday for several months. It seemed to help somewhat in the beginning but soon stalled. Then I dropped it.

*

I was hopeless and my mind was muddled but I plowed on. Somewhere in back of my mind I had a sense that I must live and raise this kid myself. For what would happen to her if I was gone? I knew I couldn't allow myself to die. I resolved to raise my little girl the best way I possibly could. I went to the library, checked out self help books and started to read them. My first pick was Dr. Mandell's 5 Day Allergy Relief.

Gradually, I got interested in gardening and producing my own fresh food without using pesticide. I began to think that was a great idea. One day I brought 4 plastic tubs home. My mother asked me what they were for. I told her I wanted to learn growing some vegetables. "That's good for nothing!" she immediately scolded me harshly. And I never got to plant anything in those boxes, eventually thrown away.

My little girl entered kindergarten and soon first grade. I found her often crying when I returned home from work and asked my mother why. It turned out that my daughter scattered things all around the floor when she played, and my mother resented cleaning up after her. She had told her, "Stop playing. Can't you sit there still?" Of course a little girl couldn't sit there still. She had to play leaving a mess.

My mother, although good at heart and so nice to others, was harsh to us her underlings. She had a harsh life and lived with her demons. Poor mother! Apparently, her devotion to God didn't help. With her dedicated church activities she built a facade of piety few can match. But her internal transformation was hard to come by. Her piety failed to melt her extreme unhappiness inside and she lived a double life.

I tried to reason with her several times but it didn't work. Eventually, I faced a difficult choice between my mother and my little daughter. I had to choose the latter for I knew well what kind of damage it did on me and was determined to end the infamous legacy in my generation. I wanted my daughter to be a clear break from the tradition and I knew I was steeped in it although I was trying to get away from it.

I told my daughter at age 9 or 10 that she's free to make all her personal decisions and told her to feel free to scream at me "if you have to." It was risky but I thought it was the only honest way to ensure that I carry out what I meant I would by giving her a say on my behavior. We had our rows and I heard quite a few of her screams during her high school years. She accused me I was controlling her and I said I wasn't. Several times I asked myself aloud, "What have I done wrong?" and took to the mountains. After a long hike I would come back with my peace. She is a mother herself of a boy and a girl, a loving, dedicated and happy mom. A clear break from my mother she is. Now back to the old days.

*

One day I called Los Angeles County – University of California Extension Services and was overjoyed to get a plot in a community garden. Although I never gardened before, I pored over gardening books at the library and planted all kinds of vegetables. My daughter loved everything I grew. She loved big old Korean squashes, picked mature as winter squashes, peeled and cut in a long string, and hung them on the guard-rail to dry. In Korea my mother used to make steamed rice cake with such dried squash pieces. I never had a chance. My daughter ate them all when half dry.

She was 11 by now. Once she brought two friends home and I offered them a fresh tomato pureed drink from tomatoes I'd grown. Her friends wouldn't touch it. I was surprised. But then I wasn't. My daughter and I, we both awoke from a happy spell we've been under. After that she wouldn't drink any more tomato drinks. But those were the heady days. Organic Gardening was a magazine I read cover to cover.*

* It was a wonderful magazine riding the tide of swelling readership attracted by the organic solutions and tired of chemical sales pitch. After the death of Robert Rodale, who brought the magazine his father started to a new high, the new management headed by his widow approved to take advertising from the chemical industry starting with the treated wood for bordering the raised garden in the name of broadening its appeal. It provoked an immediate controversy. The management ignored it. Disenchanted readers abandoned the magazine by droves, me one of them. A once unassailable first-rate publication quickly lost its steam as it was reduced struggling for survival losing its exalted place to Mother Earth

News. Now we live in different times. The Mother Earth News used the same kind of logic and pulled "broadening its readership." Apparently, this suggests their readership may be just as ambivalent as the rest of general public now.

Soon I turned to mountains topped by trees sporting the same color as my garden. They were beckoning me and I responded. I started hiking. When I started hiking at the Griffith Park in Los Angeles, I could barely walk slowly because my stomach was churning and nauseating. But I wanted to live and kept on. I went back there every Saturday and Sunday. Gradually, I sensed that I felt better after a good hike.

On Sunday, January Second, 1994 I was hiking at the Griffith Park in Los Angeles. I stopped to take a break and sat on the ground. But, lo! Something was there! A piece of dirt was broken off and being lifted. Stooping I looked closer to see what was the matter. A teeny-weeny yellow thing crooked at its neck by the weight was pushing up valiantly. I soon found out it was a wild mustard seed sprouting!

A flash of lightening ran through my head. I understood at that instant – everything! Everything about my life! A veil was lifted from my eyes! It must have been a ton of weight for the little thing! I figured it out that I was gigantic and enormously more powerful in comparison.

"Oh! Yea! If you can do it I can do it, too!" exclaimed I. All my personal problems, large and small, were instantly rendered solvable! I could make out meandering paths of my life all laid out as if looking down the field from a mountain top. Thank you, little sprout! I felt so free! An intense warm glow of euphoria with a sense of empowerment washed over me. No longer powerless or clueless, I felt confident. As time wore on, however, the clear picture, the luminous halo, the sweet juice diminished. But I knew I was a changed man now.

Then somebody told me about a waterfall in San Bernardino Mountains. "A waterfall?! In Southern California! Impossible!" I thought. I had lived there for years but never explored the mountains. A waterfall in summer in Los Angeles sounded so incredible and as much enticing. One day I drove up the hills and hiked down to the Sturdevant Falls. I was happily proved wrong. It was so exhilarating! Wow! Heaven!

One evening on a moonlight hiking I met a lady named Laura Sandiford. She invited me to a Sunday hike with her group called *Hikercize*. I joined the group and soon became one of the earnest members. At first my legs hurt and my breath was short. Yet I returned every Sunday. In about 10 years I became one of the hardiest hikers and most of my health problems disappeared except my stuffed up sinuses and muffled hearing.

A few months before I'd signed up for acupuncture school I'd written the following as part of my 4-page self affirmation statement:

I am a happy man.
I am relaxed.
I am totally relaxed.
Peace, calm, equanimity,
Boundless energy and joy are all mine here and now.

I am totally convinced truly to the core of my being
That there is nothing I could not possibly achieve
If I worked hard at it consistently and persistently.

My mind and body are healthy and strong
And maintain their integrity at all times.
Everything in my system from head to toes
Works in perfect condition and harmony.

My brain, left and right,
Spinal chords and the entire nervous system,
Meridians, and other energy channels,
Chakras, glands, internal organs,
Bones, joints, muscles,
Blood, lymph and their vessels,
Skin, hair, sexual organs,
Tissues and cells large and small,
All work in perfect condition and harmony.

Especially my once injured leg, arms and chest,
My sometimes-ulcerous stomach and its associated organs
Are flooded with healing energy day and night
And getting better every minute.

My sinus, nose, throat,
And all the cavities in the head
Including the ear canals and the tear channels
Are finally completely clear
And free of all infections, inflammations,
Swellings, and all pathogenic influences,

And are constantly patrolled by health giving fluids.

My asthma is gone, gone forever and never to return.
So are coughing, wheezing, sneezing,
And difficulty of breathing.

My whole system is rejuvenating.
My heart beats stronger,
And my energy is rising day by day.

My hair is turning black
And its sheen and luster are coming back.
My skin is tightening up firm and bouncy
Over the entire expanse of my body.

My senses are quicker and keener.
My vision is clear and sharply defined.
My hearing and smelling are fully restored
Along the full spectrum of each.
My memory and mental power stay sharp and resourceful.
Etc., etc. (Cut and omitted)

Soon after writing my self-affirmation statement shown above, in my mid-50's, I enrolled in an acupuncture school in Los Angeles and I certainly hoped I would get rid of these persistent problems someday. I had trouble in following the discussions in my classes and asked my doctor at UCLA for help. He sent me to an audiologist for a hearing test. The audiologist recommended a surgery to install a stent to help drainage from my ears and to have hearing aids fitted afterwards. Then I asked her about any risks of the surgery. She told me there was a "slight risk on vision." That turned me off immediately and strongly so. Thanks but no thanks!

I told my doctor the risk was not acceptable to me and asked for "medical help" meaning something without surgery and hearing aids. My doctor just kept mum. No word came out of his mouth. So I said thank you and had to leave. To myself I said, "I'll find a way."

Of course, I turned to my school clinic and most of my acupuncturist teachers who doubled as clinical supervisors. But nothing helped. They all explained saying, "This is a dampness problem. Dampness is stubborn, most difficult to resolve, if not impossible." And that was it.

In retrospect after all my firsthand experiences so far, I realize

regrettably now that no practitioner of the Eastern Medicine has helped me successfully overcome this stubborn so-called dampness problem. My own personal experience detailing in this book, however, using permanent lifetime dietary supplement of the very Yin Essence foods of taken in various forms in my food such as whole flax seed meal, whole almond meal, et cetera, all characterized by slippery and sticky texture when combined with water. After 6-7-8 years of continuing dietary experiment turned into permanently adopted new lifestyle choice started March 2012 and continuing through the end of my life as intended, has proven so far has given me protection over the disease that tormented me nearly 50 years.

Now I am fully convinced that Mother Nature has had full lifetime health protection over us all humans via dietary measure of slippery and sticky stuff from various source foods I name and describe throughout. Mother Earth feeds us and protects us for our good health. And this is how humanity has survived over the millennia until today. Please consider to realize and understand this. Food security and good health, these two are the cornerstone on which our life on earth is built. That's a fact that is perennially true. It is true to everyone and every human being on earth.

I graduated, got licensed and opened a practice. I wanted to help people feel better. That was my overriding goal. Can I do that? On the surface of my mind I was sure of that. But in the back I heard a former classmate teasing me, saying, "Doctor, heal thyself first!"

Listening to what a patient has to say is a critical part in the practice of Oriental medicine and I struggled with it due to my hearing difficulty especially with the soft spoken. After 7 years of practice I left California and settled at Black Mountain, North Carolina hoping to have a quiet life near the mountains while having a small practice.

I was sorry to discover my California license wasn't accepted in North Carolina and I had to jump the hoops all over again. I had to take 4 licensing exams: 1) Foundations of Oriental medicine, 2) Acupuncture, 3) Oriental herbal medicine, and 4) Biomedicine. I passed all of them at the first take but the whole process took me nearly 2 years. By the way I had ample spare time on my hand.

I focused on healing myself in earnest with a greater concentration this time on my 'permanent head cold' and hopefully to hear better. It has been 30 years — there may have been slight ups and downs, but the bottom line was unchanged. My head was basically stuffed up.

All the cranial sinuses in my head were full of mucus, or at least I felt that way. When I spoke my head didn't sound like a resonant drum but a solid rock. In my head I could sense a faint metallic trill that sent a sharp chill down my spine every time I spoke. It made a reserved man a recluse. Everybody asked me if I had a cold because they could recognize my nasal tone. My stock answer was, "No, I've got allergy. No cold." And how embarrassed I was about my deafness! I contrived, often unsuccessfully I guess, not to let the people know about my problem. Often, I couldn't follow the conversation. I wasn't very good in lip reading either. Sometimes I pretended I understood them. How risky!

*

As a result of focusing on my health I had several happy years in North Carolina, which prompted me to write the following paragraphs:

Now I am happy to announce all that crap is in the past. My head cold has completely cleared up. At my mid-60's I've got my hearing back. No surgery, no drainage stent installed, no hearing aids fitted, but naturally, I've got my hearing back 100 percent finally in my mid 60's. This is no fluke. I envisioned a complete healing more than 10 years ago, planned, worked relentlessly and finally succeeded in my mid 60's.

First time in long years I could whistle. When I tried to whistle before the sound fizzled on my lips. I didn't know why. Now I whistle freely. I used to love singing but it was difficult because of the discomforts. But now I sing freely. My head resonates like a hollow drum. I've never felt better, never felt healthier, and never felt stronger than I am now.

I apparently gloated prematurely and this euphoria was short-lived while I stayed in North Carolina.

In the ensuing years as I moved back to Korea after living nearly four decades in the U.S. I had to make a great deal of adjustments.

And as I settled in a farming village close to a seafront, about 12 miles from where I was born and grew up, I made an effort to strengthen my Yin and Jing and I thought it might be working. The most striking improvement was my easy to sunburn skin withstood intense direct sunshine on my bare shoulders. In spite of direct exposure for hours to a day as I worked in the garden my skin just tanned dark and there were no blisters, widespread reddened burn or pain. My hairline once far receded in the temples has largely grown back forward, and once wispy thin hair locks became thicker and more numerous. I was surprised and happy, which was brief, though. "Was this a true improvement that could have lasted but abruptly stalled due to the tick bite?" I am left wondering.

Chapter 6

THOROUGHLY TO OUR BONES WE ARE NATURE'S CHILDREN

For verily I say unto you
If ye have faith as a grain of mustard seed,
Ye shall say unto this mountain,
Remove hence to your place and it shall remove:
And nothing shall be impossible unto you.
St. Matthew 17:20

Because nature has made us we need to live in a nature ordained way if we wanted to stay healthy. This is a self-evident truth to my simple intellect, and it needs no further proof as far as I'm concerned. The only trouble is what it is really the nature ordained way can be uncertain in practical terms for most everybody, and I wanted to find that out and clarify it.

I had already made up my mind that whenever I needed help on my health, I would search for it from foods or herbs that are widely available to the general public at a reasonable price, with emphasis on very low price if at all possible and easy accessibility. Simply put, cheap and easy are the two operating words in my search as long as effective. The decision was also derived from my simple logic that human physiology should have been developed from eating widely available foods in the nature anyone could access to them. This led me to look into possibilities that one can grow some plants at their homes that are not widely available in current societies but once they were or had been. It was also one of my important objectives to encourage nature friendly lifestyle to my readers for there is no better way to be acquainted with the way nature works than to grow some plants and use them for food and healing.

The Main Health Problems I Faced Then

Approaching my 72nd birthday in the year 2012 while living in South Korea, I had three major health problems and a number of smaller but intractable conditions that wouldn't easily go away, although I had no real physical limitations to keep me from pursuing my active lifestyle. I will tell you about them first now in some detail before I enter discussions on my explorations into food medicine in an effort to heal my health problems through foods and foods alone and no medical treatments and not even herbs of Oriental Medicine which was a part of my professional working areas. These were my current problems at the time when I started my explorations into food medicine. Later, I would report to you on how I went along with them.

The Main Health Problems I faced in the Year 2012:

1) **Tick Bite and What I considered Its Aftermath** What I feared it to be Lyme disease in the beginning was giving me continuous crops of large red, extremely itchy rashes all over my body except my forearm, hands, feet and face, which allowed me to keep the problem secret even from my mother who lived with me on my care. They appeared sometime after I got bitten by a tick in early spring in 2011. Naturally concerned about it, I searched Internet for something to address it effectively.

(**Note:** Scared by Lyme disease stories in the U.S., I was probably overly sensitive of potential complications due to tick bites in Korea. Luckily, none of my fears materialized as of 6/13/18.)

2) **Chronic Nasal Congestion over Five Decades** My chronic nemesis ever since my early 30's, sinus congestion was still bothering me sometimes worse other times better for 5th decades of my life. One of my brothers urged me to get surgery telling me he had it done and has enjoyed with no problem since. I told him that I will take care of it my way and was determined to find a natural and permanent solution on my own. Over the years, I used all kinds of methods to stay on top of it. Some of them helped for a number of years and led me to believe as if I got rid of it for good. But the relief proved to be temporary and the nemesis always managed to come back, and I was still working on it.

(Note: Hurrah!!! I finally defeated my 50 years-old nemesis with my own fists and not by any sword, meaning that I defeated my

chronic disease only by means of food but without any kind of medicine whatsoever. Food and water alone! As of 6/13/18. Complete details in the last Chapter Eight.

3) **In-Sleep Saliva Failure Resulting in Completely Dried Mouth Stuck Shut** These words fairly well describe the first incidence of its kind I experienced. This condition first happened 6-7 years ago. In the middle of night, I was suddenly made aware of my mouth so extremely dry that my gums, cheeks, lips and tongue, all got stuck like one solid piece, unable to open the mouth and extremely uncomfortable. In the beginning the condition quickly disappeared as soon as I opened my eyes and saliva started to flow immediately, but often it came back as soon as I fell asleep. Over the years the symptoms moderated somewhat, and in summer in 2011 my concerns got considerably eased when I noticed my bare shoulders and back working the blazing sun did not burn and blister as they always did in previous years as far as I could remember. Which led me believe I was progressing in my fight against Yin Deficiency, a global term that would have included my dry mouth debacles, emaciated body, premature grey, incessant dandruff and itchy scalp and that signature pea sized red dot at the tip of my tongue. (Note: This was also solved and became a non-issue as of 6/13/18. More details in the last chapter.)

And the stubborn nature of my sinus troubles may have their roots in this Yin Deficiency, too. Therefore, I have been long concerned about my need to strengthen my Yin in back of my mind but never got seriously focused on tackling it, while I hiked aggressively for a number of years, which might have further stressed the Yin of my body. Now I'm paying my price. So, I chose to take it head on as the second phase of my food medicine exploration for the first time. I tentatively considered this problem of mine was traced back all the way to my childhood malnutrition.

Saliva Failure/Stuck Mouth is obviously pertaining to Yin problem as the term is understood in Oriental Medicine. Yin is most often understood as roughly equivalent to water and various body fluids in a narrow sense of the term. In a broader sense, however, anything that constitutes a living body except the life force itself should be called Yin including blood. The life force represents the energy that enables body to be living, called Yuan Qi in Chinese or literally translated Original Qi in English. So, all the structural components of the body, including internal organs, bones, muscles, skin, hair, nails, etc. are viewed as Yin. Blood is considered more Yin than Yang or Energy and yet more Yang than all the rest of the living body's structural components. So Blood sits in between Yin and Yang as partly Yin and partly Yang.

Now what was the nature of my Yin problem? I already said it was Yin Deficiency. The typical disharmony of Yin Deficiency is so called Deficient Heat. It often manifests as a low-grade fever and infection that usually is aggravated in the afternoon and through the night. This can be also coupled with concomitant external chills. For example, I suffered a lot from January through December in 2013 that I was practically scared to go to bed in the night. In the evening hours I began to feel feverish chills and craved warmth, but I was prevented from turning up the heat in the bedroom or using heavy comforters in fear of severe Heat/Dryness attacks once I fell asleep. I felt the warmer condition comforting before I fell asleep but the warmer and more comfortable I made myself I would experience the more severe Heat/Dryness attack later once I fell asleep. So, it was not a viable option to make myself warm and comfortable in bed. Heat/Dryness attack always occurred in the bed while I was sleeping only. I was awakened by severe *Saliva Failure/Stuck Mouth* 3 to 4 times during 6 to 8 hours of sleep every night with a few exceptions. Each time I had to pee and drink a full cup of water or two then slip back into bed and tried to sleep while at the same time I tried not to fall asleep fearing its consequences. At first, I had to drink only the warm water because as soon as I drank unheated water I had to pee again immediately. My body seemed unable to retain the water in spite of the intense Dryness I could witness all over my body. Especially my forearms and lower legs were shriveled dry and practically reduced to bones and sickly creased skins. My muscles in the chest, biceps in the upper arms and the calves all shrunk away leaving the skin creased like an old drapery. It was truly depressing. Some nights more severe and other nights slightly less so, but the pattern repeated every night. During the day I aggressively drank water in hope to reduce nighttime Dryness but the effort had absolutely no effect at all. Only thing it did was swell my legs and feet with edema during the waking hours, which will be drained completely in the night leaving the depressing sight again of the bone and skin of the night before.

(Note: The scary descriptions in Saliva Failure/ Stuck Mouth given above were my personal experiences through one winter-and-spring while living in Korea and never repeated thereafter. As of 12/15/18 I am relieved to find the various drying experience episodes described above turned out to be temporary adjustments.)

At first, I was really distressed about my miserable state of Yin, but it slowly dawned on me that it was a process that was in passing

somehow due to my continued twice daily ingestion of mucilaginous fiber since March 2012, which had the power of attracting 1,000 times its dry weight of water.

The above three were my major health threats I was facing. I might add that anyone of them was serious enough to qualify me for a lifetime clinical care as I get older. **But I was determined to keep them off just by eating and drinking my daily fare of foods and water. And that's what I did and am committed to continuing to do so until my last day.**

The First Phase of My Search
From March through December 2012
I pondered long and hard how to fight my health woes, a few and relatively small but at the same time very persistent and aggravating. I also considered I was at my early 70's and these woes are likely to deepen as I get older unless I found the ways to deal with them successfully and may be the one that eventually may take me under if not. I thought about how frustrating it would be if I was left struggling to breathe gasping for the air with my airways helplessly blocked. And I didn't wish to end up in a hospital hooked up with breathing tubes. So, I had to find ways to help me out on my own. And that's exactly what I decided to do.

I also decided my chief means to achieve that goal had to be following the dictum of Hippocrates and teachings of the Oriental medicine in self nurturance. Although the self-nurturance practices in China and Korea use the herbs of the traditional medicine quite liberally, I decided not to use any herbs of professional medicine unless it was cheap and widely available to the consumer at the grocery ails in the United States. That leaves out most of the medicinal herbs of the Oriental medicine. I am eagerly anticipating, though, planting the seeds of one Chinese herb called jiaogulan (Gynostemma pentaphyllum) in Chinese and obtaining its leaves to make tea. Although long used in southern China as an "Immortality Herb" this native Chinese herb has recently emerged from its relative obscurity promising to be a top flying and one of the most popular herbs in the world. (Yes, I fantasized this herb from southern China as an ideal tea making herb, bought a plant by mail and grew it at home in dry climate of Northern California. After one year I regrettably decided that the plant will only thrive in a warm moisture rich environment and I had to give it up. I had to find another more mundane solution for moisturizing my throat as I will tell you later.)

A year later now, however, I find a renewed interest in growing jiaogulan for tea herb and entertaining the thought of sipping the tea brewed out of that herb. I'll see in the spring. Maybe!

Self-Care Is the Necessary and Firm Foundation to Build A Thriving Life on!!!

3E Essentials for Your Health; that is, Eat, Exercise and Enthuse!!!

Years ago when I was asked to speak to a local senior citizens' group as a practicing acupuncturist in Glendale, California, I gave them three principles to rely on for their future health: 1) regular balanced diet, 2) regular appropriate exercises, and 3) emotional light-heartedness, and positive enthusiasm on your life. Later on I developed the idea into a succinct memorable phrase: 3 E Essentials for health, which included *EAT, EXERCISE and ENTHUSE* in which I mean I embrace my life whole-heartedly, or enthusiastically. I still abide by these principles. Therefore, while this book is mostly dedicated on the subject of *EAT*, I want to add just a paragraph each on the subjects of *EXERCISE,* right here and *ENTHUSE* , after that.

- **EXERCISE:** Man used to hunt for food in the wild or work hard long days in the fields. Now most people work all day long sitting in an office chair year after year. Apparently, therefore, we need some walking exercises, and often plenty of them. People exercising regularly maintain their bodies fit and tend to stay largely healthy. Most every community has their share of rivers, valleys, mountains, hills and fields. So I would ask the communities to parcel out some of these landscapes into some small parks and long trails to induce people regardless their skin colors, men or women, rich or poor come out often, enjoy and help themselves stay fit. Communities wildly differ in this. I lived a few years in Midlothian in Virginia, a Richmond suburb and found no small parks or trails nearby and had to walk roadside with no sidewalks twice a day, having to constantly deal with passing cars. Now moved back to Northern California with a county park and a nearly endless trail right outside of my doorstep I'm very happy most every day. It's heavenly to live here!

- **Enthuse:** "Man shall not live by bread alone but by every word that proceedeth out of the mouth of God", as Jesus was ascribed to have said. I take liberty of interpreting the phrase "out of the mouth of God" would also include people speaking "out of their hearts," for we should be allowed to speak out our hearts aloud. In the past they used to say, "Words can't hurt you." But it simply isn't so. Words can inflict serious physical harm, too. And also our ability to express what we feel inside, in plain words and not resort to angry shout outs, and not to dwell on grudges for long but to forgive, forget and move on powerfully affects not only our health but also our happiness. Simply put, it isn't worth to be tied down by grudges. And also consider reading on my next article on Original Blessing.

Chapter 7

DISCOVERING MY ROOT – THE ORIGINAL BLESSING

When I reach deep inside, I find two spiritual instincts at the root of my heart. I will call them the spirit of self-reliance and the spirit of community. They may seem to pull me to opposite directions, the former to my own self-interests and the latter to the others and the interests of the community. I decided to call this spiritual gift "The Original Blessing" for I strongly believed in it and in part in defiance and rejection of the dogma of the Original Sin of the Catholic Church. This unfortunate, what I consider to be based on a fairy tale, helped the church to enslave millions of souls in the guilt that they are not responsible for and control their lives to this day. Now the humanity has the full truth and is entitled to take advantage of making The Original Blessing firmly established in their hearts and liberate themselves in the spirit of self-reliance and the spirit of community. The twin spirit is not of two but one whole and undivided. This represents the true born nature of every human being.

The spirit of self-reliance enables me to discover my true self, and to value and love myself. It also empowers me to pursue my potentials. I see the seed or budding root of this spirit in my grandchildren and any babies when they try to spoon themselves, want to do everything their way and on their own, in which they take pride and joy. We must recognize this and encourage it so that each of them has a chance to bloom into becoming a fully self-competent individual independent of their parents eventually. In the past adults often emphasized their authority and demanded obedience by children unilaterally. I grew up with the dictum that said: a man's word is worth one thousand pieces of gold encouraging us to keep the mouth shut.

This is the source from which my sense of dignity, individuality, self-esteem and self-confidence come. I may be fragile, but these qualities make me strong. When parents love a child, care for its needs, and properly nurture its self-expression, the child blooms into an able self-reliant and creditable member of the society. On the other hand, when the parent fails, the child is at risk of falling to wimpy self-doubt, cynicism, or, if abused, violent rebellion to the society.*

*For more information on how early childhood shapes the later adult life, but fortunately, that this is not fixed for life and can be changed by mental training due to brain plasticity and one's life can be transformed, read Chapter 8 "Blaming Mom? Rewired for Compassion," in Sharon Begley's book, *Train Your Mind, Change Your Brain, How a New Science Reveals Our Extraordinary Potential to Transform Ourselves,* © 2007, Ballentine Books, New York.

In my case, I fell as a victim to a severe and prolonged self-doubt, deprived of my self-confidence and left out in an abyss of fogged confusion. I see now that the confusion was a result of suspended judgment on my part whether to break through the opposition to assert myself or cowered by my Mother and obey her absolutely. Apparently, I couldn't choose either way or carve out my own way somewhere in the middle.

So my heart got caught in limbo between its desire and the opposition it met and was left dangling in between through much of my whole lifetime. Why I was so serious and couldn't have used some humor or something and wiggle out of that tight space while growing up I do not know. So I do know from my firsthand experience how vulnerable a child's spirit can be and how critically important it is to nurture it.

This history may still leave me perhaps one slight chance at becoming a so-called late bloomer. It remains to be seen.

* The Spirit of Community, a more subtle counterpart of the spirit of self-reliance, may seem less assertive, but is just as deeply rooted in us. A child is born of a social relationship of a man and a woman. He or she is nurtured and cared for by, and begins his/her earthly journey, with his/her parents and the others around them. You can

notice how even young children love to help their parents notwithstanding their limited abilities and often unable to help than hinder, but still they take pride in being allowed to help. Is this tendency some kind of seed and budding root of something, too, if encouraged, can materialize into really big years later? I tend to think so, and that's why I want to call it The Spirit of Community.

In the course of growing up the child watches parents and the others and learns socializing with them earning their approval, securing a comfortable place for himself/herself in the community and rising to being a useful and creditable member to benefit his/her community.

Every day when I walk through the nearby County Park, I often come across to witness precious moments of young children communicating with their parents, some blurt outs here and there, scenes of some toddlers of different sizes pushing their own sizes of roller skates, or even younger kid being pushed in a baby buggy often intently staring into his or her hand-held phone equivalent devices. All these show me tidbits of pleasure and reward of raising the crop of our next generation.

Both the Spirit of Self Reliance and the Spirit of Community may be the two expressions of the same cause: securing a comfortable place for oneself. While the former is narrowly focused on self and the latter represents an expanded view of self to be inclusive of his fellow human beings. One's personal growth with strong relationships with the community strengthens own security as well as advances the community interests.

Balancing one's self interests against those of others is apt to turn out in the long run to be an enlightened pursuit of self-interests as I believe Abraham Lincoln personifies. This way one becomes a balanced whole being, and both of his selfish and altruistic forces are expressed and melt in a compromise dissolving conflicts. It is my personal goal to have my spirit of individual self-reliance be well balanced against my spirit of community solidarity at all times and I recommend a similar goal to you. I believe we all share a basic willingness to help when we see someone struggling. But our world is full of contradictions, which I cannot deny. Ultimately, it's up to the conscious choices, yours as well as mine, trying to engage both sides of our spiritual inheritance and end up in a somewhat balanced way.

This is the very source of physical as well as mental health and the sometimes-elusive thing that is called happiness comes from. How do I pursue my dream and be one with the universe at the same time? I think just by being true to my deeper self and natural instincts, as apparently epitomized in nature by the triplets* of the trees I found on Vermont Canyon in Los Angeles and the millions of barley stalks in my father's old barley fields** I watched in my childhood wondering how densely they stood to each other and how well each of them did. When I reflect on those childhood recollections I can't but wonder into how distant past the origin of The Original Blessing may be traced back – perhaps into pre-pre-primordial times.

The spirit of self-reliance
And the spirit of the community
Are like the two wings of a bird.
If we have them both strong
We can soar up high into the sky.

Likewise, we humans can protect and maintain our health indefinitely by the natural means available to everybody, rich or poor, if we are aware and motivated enough to do the right things to protect ourselves because the Mother Nature is on our side. As long as we work and can put foods on the table and follow my suggestion on proper hydration, our health can be protected and maintained indefinitely. We have been put in the dark so long as to what the nature's contribution to the humanity's health can be so that many of us have forgotten how to properly care for ourselves to maintain our health and strength by our own self-care, and more seriously so in our younger generations. The ability to enjoy the security both in foods and health can be a great equalizer in our society, where an extreme inequality is the rule now and generates extreme conflicts. With these two things securely taken care of, each of us can go out and compete freely and fairly to bring out what is the best in each of us.

The illuminated sense of empowered self as an individual and a member of the community can be the cornerstone leading to the realization of justice for all democratic society along with the security in health attained largely through the means of self-care based on Mother Nature's protection. I believe we individuals have the capacity to work together for common goals.

*If you visited Los Angeles and hopefully the Greek Theatre and the Observatory, you would have passed by but surely missed the three trees planted close to each other in the middle of the road, grew to good mature tree sizes and beautifully compromised in sharing the air spaces equitably between themselves and presenting a beautifully well-balanced canopy for themselves.

****I have a distinct memory in my childhood of how beautifully shining were the densely standing barley stalks drenched in spring sunlight when I was chasing a pheasant mother and her chicks perhaps about a dozen of them passing through the barley stalks expertly and disappearing soon into nowhere.**

I Loved the Market Day Street Fair in Korea
Most Fish and Sea Greens I Miss in the U.S.

In combating my health woes and protecting it beyond, I decided to use exclusively the common foods that are available at the market at reasonable prices. Because I was living in a southern coastal area in South Korea most of my foodstuff was coming from local sources. A great variety of fishes, clams, squids, sea greens, vegetables such as napa cabbage, a variety of radishes, spinach, soybean sprouts, mung bean sprout, etc., etc., all aplenty on every market day that comes every 5th day, displayed in the middle of the road, where all the vehicular traffic was temporarily blocked, most fish and some vegetables were often trimmed and cleaned by the hard working farmers' wives and street peddlers for the convenience of the buyer. Prices were reasonable and foodstuff was fresh with large crowds from dense population eager to buy. Sometimes you find an unusual thing or two. It was a fun place to visit. I loved to go on marketing most every 5 or 10 days. That's one thing I really miss after returning to the U.S. In this country only some farmers' markets may offer somewhat similar atmosphere, although in a very limited sense.

My favorite fishes were mainly those caught fresh by local fishermen in the nearby coastal region such as Pacific mackerels, sardines, anchovies, eels, squids, oysters, shrimps, crabs, octopus, various shell fishes, etc., as well as various fresh sea greens in the fall through early spring, and some imported fishes such as pollack in the Russian waters, and sometimes frozen prawns from Malaysian waters in the South Asian region. Although I hesitated to consume so many fish out of concern of mercury poisoning at first, I soon set it aside, joined the crowds and welcomed them into my diet. I looked for various smaller fishes which have shorter life spans and therefore less exposure to contamination. These smaller fishes, shrimps, crabs, etc., along with various seaweeds may have been humanity's earliest and most accessible food sources, and possibly among the healthiest. Although many in the U.S. still deny global warming, many of my favorite cold-water fishes once plentiful along the Korean East Coast when I was growing up such as cod, pollack, and herring are no longer found there and all of them now completely migrated north to the Russian waters or into the Arctic Region as the warm water of the Tropical Region pushed upward.

On the other hand, I had trouble in buying some of my food items while staying in Korea. Chief among them was rice because I wanted organically grown brown rice, but Korean markets didn't have them. Although I was considerably less dependent on it than most of my Korean cousins the rice was still the anchor of my diet. The only organically grown rice in Korea would be the Australian imports of long grain, they told me, but there were no outlets carrying it in my area, and even if I could get it somehow my mother wouldn't take it. So, I had to settle on regular medium grain brown rice. For most Koreans, medium grain polished white rice was the only thing they would be willing to eat. Besides, when I wanted some fermented dairy products, there was nothing available to please my taste. Even what was marked as plain yogurt there was sugar in it. There was no real butter or cheese. What they labeled as butter or cheese was adulterated by half of solidified soy oil and added color to make it look like cheddar cheese or butter.

I bought some black rice at a price of two and half times the regular rice, and some black and red beans for their antioxidant values. I could also buy some sorghum, which I valued highly about its potential antioxidant power. It was imported from China. They have a long tradition in southern China of producing high alcohol distilled liquor with more than 50% alcohol through repeated fermentation. Maotai is the most famous brand of it. There seem to be many other distilleries. I bought some small bottles of it under several different names in Korea recently as well as in the U.S. several years ago. The liquor is claimed to have high antioxidant power. Only other liquor to offer this antioxidant power in my experience was tequila brewed 100% from maguey leaves, although in the west brandy is known but I would think it would be way behind. So, I was very positive about sorghum and I wasn't disappointed. I used one third sorghum in my mixed grain and beans dish, which I simply refer to it as "rice". I enjoyed it as an ingredient in my mixed grain, beans and nuts 'rice' pot very much while living in Korea. Now that I'm tucked in mountainous wild central Virginia, I'm cutoff from sources of it and unable to put my hands on some. I'm pretty sure, though, if I had a chance to visit New York or Los Angeles I could locate some in a Middle Eastern or African community.

About 5 years later now in 2016 when I moved to Los Gatos near so called Silicone Valley in Northern California, I have wider choices and most anything I would dream of eating. The mixed rice and beans I have recently adopted are long grain red rice from Thailand, red sorghum, and red kidney beans. So, they are all red. One cup each and three cups cooked together, to be held in the fridge and about a small cupful is added to one-pot meal and re-cooked each time twice a day. The main ingredients of the one-pot meal are: a chunk of frozen fish (usually sockeye salmon in the morning), a thin slice of tofu, a half of golden beet root sliced, soaked seaweed in 1/2 cup of water, 1 tablespoonful of blanched almond flour, and 2 flat teaspoonfuls of raw cocoa nibs. And in the evening, I use a little frozen chunk of what is known as chicken tenders as my main protein source food. In the last couple of years, I preferred fattening slices of bacon, skirt steak or flat steak, and got fattened up, and I wanted stop fattening. I find it a bit challenging but I'm trying.

The resulting 'rice' pot from all these mixtures of grains, colored beans, and nuts as I added later like filberts, almonds, pumpkin seeds and sometimes chestnuts, looked exactly like the traditional meal called "medicinal rice" eaten in celebration of the First Full Moon of the Lunar New Year. It opened my eyes to realize, that my Korean ancestors must have started this holiday with a vision assuring of future popular health, and that somehow, they knew the health promoting qualities those various ingredients possessed.

In a typical Korean meal, a bowl of rice is always considered the indispensable main part and the rest were considered Banchan or side dishes. Normally you see several side dishes accompanying your bowl of rice, but in my simple and sparse lifestyle I had usually only one side dish, which was soup or salad. Occasionally, I might have one or a few side dishes except the soup or salad, cooked and seasoned vegetables or namul in Korean when either I bought some or a visitor brought me some. Occasionally I made some namul but rarely repeated to make them except once or twice. Mostly I threw everything either in my soup pot or in my salad bowl because that was easier and simpler. I used to make quite a bit of side dishes while my daughter was growing up but once she left home for college my cooking mode got simplified. And a bowl of rice and another bowl of soup or salad has become the rule ever since.

I tended to have soup when the weather was cold and salad when the weather became warm. When my attention was on making a soup for my anti-inflammatory diet I chose a popular Korean recipe of maeuntang or Hot Spicy Soup. The major ingredients called for in this soup are a goodly chunk of a fish, a tiny token slice of beef or pork, a few vegetables, some shellfish, hot pepper powder or fermented hot pepper sauce for both color and spice, a spicy green pepper or two chopped in, green onion and garlic. Usually, the most popular fish in this soup is the croaker from the west coast Yellow Sea but my choice was Pacific sardines or mackerel for its high omega 3 fatty acids. Among the vegetables I used a large chunk of giant Korean radish sliced thin and into bite sizes.

I used this soup until December 2012 but from January next year I had to quit this hot soup because of nighttime dry mouth became serious. At the same time, I banned all spicy foods, even the non-spicy bell pepper, which was spicy to my tongue, anything that is volatile, draining or drying, including all the spices and fragrant things such as citrus fruit, coffee and alcohol. Sometime in early 2018 I looked for and found an Indian grocer and bought 3 little packages (200g each) of turmeric powder, which yields deep dark yellow coloring, Kasmiri chili powder with nice warm color but with just a very, very mild hint of the spiciness, (later changed for still less spicy, but visually more redness with "Crushed Chili powder" that includes lots of seeds), and Methi Bhardo or crushed Fenugreek seeds, because my usual Korean spices became too spicy for me I wanted to find something less spicy from a long traditional culture. That's how I chose the combination. It gave me right balance and now I came to love it. Recently I made some hard to chew kimchi with dakuan radish tubers with green tops, a second time yesterday, and found it very helpful in fighting against the dementia pressures I have been under. I later changed to the short stompy type of radishes favored by Koreans, called chong-gak-muu. These are some new territories I have been forced to explore in an effort to keep my memory protected, December 26, 2018. But eventually I came to rely on eating lotus seeds (6 x 2 a day) for my memory protection. I feel my memory loss is still progressing, although I am adamantly trying to protect. (May 10, 2020)

For occasional quick lunches I often enjoyed a plate of steamed chestnuts, small pieces of sweet potato, kabocha squash and an egg. This was years ago while I stayed in Korea for a few years. Now I hardly use any eggs but sweet potato and kabocha squash have become part of my standard meal plan but in very tiny slices. My meal plan has evolved quite a bit by moving around, my continued and progressing interest of simplifying my self-reliant food preparation steps and required workload, and some new steps by my recently heightened interest of memory loss prevention. Hence, I feel the need to present what my current meal plan looks like as of December 27, 2018. I use quite a bit of almond tortillas and try to use more organic whole almonds these days. May 10, 2020.

THIS IS MY CURRENT RECIPE PLAN TO DOUBLE AS MY LIFETIME HEALTH PLAN 12/27/18

My current plan is composed of several parts: Details follow.

1)   My Chewable Radish Kimchi/ Sliced Tubers and Green Tops

I am appreciative to have this fresh uprooted organically grown radish bundles. I brought out a large stainless-steel bowl and a basket so I could clean and salt them properly. I first separated the tops and the tubers and washed them separately clean. I ran a small knife along the center of the radish vertically one after another. I sliced each pair at 1/4 inch thick across into small half-moon sizes. Next, I cut the leaves at 1/2-inch lengths. And then I mixed the both tops and tuber slices more or less evenly taking care not to bruise the leaves, which may release an undesirable bruised green grass-like flavor. And then I stirred up the whole while sprinkling coarse imported salt from Korea. I used 3 heaping spoonfuls of salt on 3 bunches of radishes. I let it salt and left it alone for a whole day. The next day I brought out the large bowl again and seasoned the stuff with appropriate herbs to make kimchi, adding crushed ginger, garlic and green onions. I might also add a few of my jalapeno peppers chopped in as long as they are available on my garden plants. Salting releases some water from the vegetables. Hope it would be just right, neither too salty nor too bland. That's it.

2)   My Daily Noon Meal Plan

Ingredients: 1) I take a kabocha squash, wash it and let it dry. Then I carve out both the stem end and the blossom end of the squash fruit using a small and sharp knife carefully. This can be tricky, but I learned to do it over the years. Then I place the squash on a cutting board securely, and then take out a large kitchen knife, place it squarely across the center of the squash, and now using my both hands with gentle seesawing action and constantly straight downward pressure. As a result, the whole squash ends up split into two equal slices. I will eventually cut each half into four equal vertical halves, and in total into 8 equal halves, but I cut them only as far as needed as I go. Because each of these theoretical 8 vertical pieces will be cut further into 4 equal smaller slices, first across and then vertically, so that only one tiny 1/32 slice of a whole kabocha squash will be used for each meal, with rest of unused squash pieces stored in the refrigerator in an open plastic bag to allow some air flow to keep them from molding; 2) A silver dollar-like 1/4 inch thick slice of Chinese yam, or called 'ma' in Korean language, peeled, 3) A 1/8 vertical slice of golden beet root, 4) An inch thick slice of Korean/ Japanese sweet potato, or the purple variety when available. I further cut each of the above four into 2 equal parts and arrange them on both edges of my pot, left and right facing each other across the center. 5) Next, the center is filled first by dumping 12 hours presoaked small cut pieces of seaweed known as Dashima in Korean or confu or kunfu, or also known as sea tangle, in a half cup of water; 6) I used to buy bulk dry goods for several years but now that I don't eat as much, I used to when I was younger, so I have small amounts of left over dry goods of several kinds and I want to consume them by adding 1 or 2 Tbsp at a time. I'm now depleting my box of mung beans, the next will be kidney beans, red wild rice, and red sorghum. It will take some time to finish all these left-over dry goods. 7) Next, I take 4 frozen asparagus spears, cut them into 1-inch-long pieces and dump them over at the center area. 8) Then I take one level Tbsp of raw cocoa nibs and place them divided into two halves on top of each side of kabocha squash/ma pieces, 9) and then I take one level Tbsp of golden flaxseed meal and place half of each on top of cocoa nibs on both sides. 10) And then I take 8 pieces of ginko nuts and place them two each on 4 corners alongside the edges. Please refer to one of the photographs showing the arrangement. It simply shows how I do it. It's up to you, of course, how you would choose to do. And then I take a bunch of smaller sea foods like 8 pieces of medium sized frozen shrimps with tops removed, at the center, and a couple of handfuls of shelled shellfish around the edges. And then I take one large leaf of red/purple chard, chop it up and sprinkle over the top. And then I add 1/2 cup of water, making the total one full cup. For seasoning, I sprinkle carefully 1/4 tsp each of turmeric powder, kasmiri chili powder (later switched to "Crushed Red Pepper") and methi bhardo or crushed fenugreek seeds bought at an Indian grocer, over the whole pot. I cook the pot on gas stove at full heat the first 10 minutes, at half heat next 5 minutes and then the last 5 minutes at the lowest setting. That leaves some thickened broth by mucilage, which I appreciate. The 'ma' pieces, asparagus spears, and seaweed slices and the already mostly dissolved golden flaxseed meal represent my chosen mucilage source foods in this recipe. As I understand it these mucilage rich foods, by Mother Nature's grace, work to guarantee my health for life as I have explained earlier. Therefore, it is important that these foods are included in the every meal in my life.

3) My Daily Midnight Meal Plan

I used to take 2 identical meals per day, midday and midnight, for some time and feel like keeping it that way indefinitely except for the small change I made above on my noon meal plan. From now on my noon meal, I'll use whatever smaller sea food items I found on my previous shopping day, but for the midnight meal I'll keep using the same Trader Joe's slice of packaged sockeye salmon. And only occasionally when the salmon piece appears to be too small, I'll add a few shrimps or similar smaller sea food items. Therefore, my midnight meal will consist with 10 little items I listed above, plus one slice of sockeye salmon, topping it with chopped red/purple chard leaf and the same seasoning as stated above. Well, eventually I cut out the salmon completely, and now I prefer a variety of smaller fishes. They are all less fatty, so I decided to use Alaskan salmon oil supplement. As a result, my waistline is becoming a little loose. Now I realize that my body with its ancient wisdom prefers to hold on any excess fat at a beck and call distance just in case of a famine. So as long as a famine is not likely your midline is unlikely to shrink unless you nearly starve any fat. I learned that lesson and share it with you. This little piece of information still may be a secret to many of us.

4) I Eventually Stumbled My Way Into All Vegetarian "Happy Meal," Without Planning to.

I thought I have had so much trouble with protein especially with amino-acid lysine vs. arginine. I have had long history of inadequate lysine, which caused me frequent migraine headache and also frequent pain in lower gum tissue. My typical response has been either adding yogurt, or recently fish such as canned sockeye salmon or sardines. Recently I used good portions of my three vegetarian staples such as 1) golden beet root, 2) kabocha squash, and Korean/Japanese sweet potato, or preferably purple sweet potato when available, and a half piece slice of Trader Joe's Organic Sprouted Tofu, just to make sure. Probably that was it. Recently I could have added sometimes a handful of frozen shellfish or something, or not at all. I haven't had any migraine headache or gum tissue pain. If anything at all I could throw in a handful of clamshell fish. I think that's a happy ending to my once chronic migraine headache and/or frequent gum tissue pain. I got free from those annoying stuff in my own all vegetarian staples. Hooray!!! (6/5/20)

5) My Choices of Desert, All in Fruits

I used to enjoy small dark wine grapes and when they quickly ran out of the season, I chose some small red grapes. But I think now that I would rather plant some wine grapes myself next year and see what happens. Before trying the dried squid, I was doing fine with my deserts, but now I must keep them out. I prefer Turkish organic dried apricots and/or persimmons of non-sulfite added. Otherwise, I'll go without desert until the next season comes around. As I get older, I tend to eat less and fewer fruits. May 10, 2020.

6) My Juice Drink After Meal, with Almond Meal, or Roasted Whole Almonds to Chew on

This fantastic drink, which I started with mulberry juice and almond-coconut milk, went through quite a bit of evolution. When I first considered a juice to protect yin mulberry was my first and pomegranate juice has become my second choice. After trying both of them I found the mulberry juice too sweet for my taste and there was another consideration that the mulberry juice was quite novel in this country and may not quite fan out and soon become unavailable in this country. Then I thought that the almond as a close relative to apricot was the really the one I wanted and got rid of the addition of coconut and its additional calories and chose Organic original almond milk. Then I combined 1/3 cup pomegranate juice, 1/3 cup unsweetened original organic almond milk, and 1/3 cup plain water, repeated 4 times a day, was my primary hydration as well as healing potion along with my mucilage rich foods, that was responsible for the healing of my body from all disease conditions I have had. All the diseases have been completely wiped out and then I was bothered by some persistent itching and I finally tracked it down to my favorite drink pomegranate juice. I experimented with increased amount of almond meal and or roasted whole almond kernels. I chose in favor of chewing roasted whole almond kernels, and this decision inspired me to add whole almond kernels to my favorite old-fashioned meal as shown in number 7) below. Then I decided not to go on that path. I may keep some whole almonds as snacks but rule out any almond drink because I was sick to piling up empty containers almost as thick as wooden boxes, know nowhere to send to proper recycling, made me decide one day, "Enough! No more!" When I can't find a recycling place for these good wooden boxes in the Northern California there is no such place in the entire nation. That was when I decided to quit my favorite drink. Now I am ready to try hemp seed meal drink to replace almond milk or chewing on my pan roasted whole almonds. I chose chewing roasted whole kernel almonds. (1/21/19).

7) My Old-Fashioned Meal with Addition of Whole Almond Kernels

I have been favorably talking about the traditional meals as being the healthy choice of meals. As a child I loved my deep purple colored rice, on my birthdays, and on major holidays throughout the year. We didn't have any notion of a birthday cake while I was growing up. If there were anything approaching its equivalence it was this steaming hot bowl of deep red bean colored sweet rice, not sugar sweet but soft tender and sticky rice sweet. Now at my old age and living in the Northern California I can add anything I might favor. As I was adding years however, my traditional meal has become bit too heavy for my digestive system and I tended to be gassy. I feel increasingly sluggish, tired and loathsome to do things I used to do to feed myself and my overriding concern is to simplify things down to the minimum. Either fresh roasted on a pan to be used with my favorite drink of pomegranate juice or cooked with my traditional mix of grains and beans, the addition of whole almond kernel has been seriously considered as the crowning touch of the digestive efficiency, and I wanted to share it with my readers. The traditional caveat of beans being gassy may have thus been successfully and pleasantly overcome. I'm so very tired to continue and let someone else check out this lead. (1/21/19)

Mother Returns to Her Daughter-in-Law

Around this time, May 2012, my mother took a fall. My rooster who was let loose in my inner courtyard attacked her by jumping on her and causing her to fall flat on her face. She got a bruise on a corner of her mouth, which became swollen. We hoped that once it goes down, she would be O.K. But in a few days, she complained of pain in her low back and was unable to walk. Her 5th lumbar got crushed, the doctor told us. After 4 or 5 days in the hospital she got bored and wanted to come home. She felt fine, she said. The doctor recommended a longer stay, though. The rest of her hospital roommates were all in pitiful states and quite distressing even to look at. I thought she might be doing better at home environment and concurred in her wish to come home, which turned out to be premature. She had pain and became immobile again. We took her back to the hospital and had her stay there for another week.

While my mother was staying in the hospital, we agreed that my brother and sister-in-law would drive her to their home with them once she gets finally discharged. So on the day she got discharged I came back home alone without my mother, picked up all her personal belongings and took them to my brother's home. That's how my mother moved back in with my brother after staying for two years with me. I feel gratified that things turned out so well. I will continuously pay my attention so that this alliance will go on indefinitely. My mother herself poses the greatest risk and having her temperament and tongue in check is challenging and unpredictable. While I'm living close by I can stop by from time to time and help defuse any hard feelings smoldering from flaring up.

Once my mother is gone, I felt free to do whatever I wanted. When I first served her my brown rice-based meal, she was quite resistant to it complaining that it was hard to chew and rough on her stomach. I had explained to her that I had already addressed those issues in my rice by mixing different grains appropriately to improve its texture. Besides, the whole grains tasted better with deep and rich flavors, not to mention its higher nutritional values, while white rice was not only bland and tasteless it was deficient in nutrition, I explained patiently, and she eventually turned around and came to enjoy the full flavors of mixed grains and beans.

The history of average Korean people eating polished white rice has not been long – no more than several decades. And even the earliest date any Koreans could possibly have eaten white rice might be after 1910, when Korea was annexed by Japan. Japanese got their first milling machines from Europeans probably in the 1890's. No one could have had any white rice before this date. Besides rice was always in short supply and priced out of the reach of masses of people who had to use mainly barley, wheat, corn, potato and sweet potato with tiny amount of rice, which was reserved for the old and young, until 1980's when mechanical farming was widely adopted and as a result Korea achieved self-sufficiency in rice production. Many of the Koreans, however, are quasi-addicted to it by now. One of my former neighbors told me that he would rather die than eat brown rice. And in the early turn of the 20th century in Japan beriberi became a serious disease due to the introduction of milled white rice. My mother recalled her old memory and told me after these exchanges that she had a cousin who married a Korean man living in Japan "died young because she ate rice that we couldn't even have put our eyes on," she said.

Chapter 8

A SELF CARE PROGRAM OF ACTION TO PROTECT OUR HEALTH FOR LIFE

Mother Nature's Natural Protection Makes
Our Lifetime Self Healthcare Plan Feasible

Our life on earth as a human is not as helpless or precarious as a candlelight at the whims of a prevailing wind. Sadly, to say, however, our conscious mind can be sometimes as shifty as such a proverbial candlelight in the wind from time to time. That is our real problem. The human race, generations after generations, flourished on earth for hundreds of thousands of years, and in my opinion, on the solid protection by nature through the means of the communities faithfully adhering to the teachings of their ancestral diet. In the modern era, however, those of us living in the so called well developed and technologically advanced countries as societies diversified lost sight of the wisdom of following the traditional diet of our ancestors. What we don't realize is, this change or neglect rather, turned the nature's age-old protection often untenable by rendering the key nutrient that is the mucilage out of reach of our young folks who prefer white bread and white rice but dislike the rough outer part of the grains or any other roughages that will supply them the nutrients they missed in white bread and white rice. The mucilage is also known as soluble fiber, or "viscous and elastic substances," a term that is preferred by some scientists, or "sticky and slippery stuff," a thickening agent better known in Cajun diet, and a term commonly understood among ordinary people describing the juicy inner bark of broken branch of an American elm tree, for example. But among the devotees of the traditional eastern medicine in China and the Orient, this substance was largely known as Yin, a term often used in a phrase that goes: "Yin equals water," or sometimes was called more precisely as Yin Essence. I do not know how far these terms, Yin or Yin

Essence goes back in history, but at least 2,000 years may be a reasonable guess. Anyway, note that this term Yin was used as tautological to water. I got a hint from this usage and perceived to find the traditional term Yin and a relatively modern English term "mucilage" identical and to be essential and indispensable nutritional substance needed to change the water obtained from nature into body fluid, and therefore essential and indispensable nutritional substance for proper hydration. In my opinion, the proper hydration provides the nature's ultimate human race health protection for life as long as one continues consuming this substance, which is strongly anti-inflammatory. It is my inference that few, if any at all, individuals in the past may have consumed this mucilage thing consciously, but I assume enough of it was almost always included in the foods they ate most every day in their life, as long as they adhered to what they considered to be their ancestral traditional foods. This is the conclusion of my personal study of mucilage rich food items, which I started in March 2012 while living in Korea for a few years, then moved back to the States living a few years in Virginia, and finally to Los Gatos, in Northern California, and all along continuing my study, which spanned over 7 years as of now 6/19/18. And in April 2020, I moved again to San Clemente, in Orange County in Southern California. Hereby I mean the nature has a solid and unfailing plan to protect our health for our lifetime as long as we get continuous supply of this nutrient, the Yin Essence, or mucilage through our lifetime as long as we adhere to our ancestral food. But in these modern and diversified societies in which we live everything depends on our conscious decisions most every day.

The Balance Ensures Freedom from Disease and Pain

The central most important point in consideration of my dietary choices is always on maintaining the balance. The balance between Yin foods and Yang foods is responsible for keeping the body *free from disease* and *free from pain.* Once again, by Yin Foods I mean mucilage, water and roughages, and by Yang Foods, I mean all the calorie producing foods such as protein, carbohydrates and lipids. I am here to demystify the issues of our health. In my understanding, *the nature's scheme in protecting us humans to stay healthy is simple, uncomplicated and natural!* And that's how our human race was brought up by nature until today. So, we must keep in our mind always – it's in our best interest to keep it simple as nature taught us. Let's look for a simple balance in most every meal, day in and day out. *A good balance means any inflammatory pressure is brought down to zero or non-existent, which means, always or today, tomorrow, and every day.* As long as this state prevails no disease or pain will occur. Is it possible then to maintain this balance indefinitely or for one's whole lifetime? My answer to this question is an unreserved yes! And absolutely! *So, let's get resolved to keep it that way.* If you happen to be in a long and serious disease and pain, you can consult your health professional about starting this balancing diet. The following represents food sources I tried interchangeably over 7+ years and proved personally safe and effective for the purpose. I pray that you have confidence to try and see through it all the way. In case you are overweight and decide to cut back calories, be sure to work with your health professional and proceed slowly but surely over a few to several years.

Here is a caution to you. I am absolutely sure of what I say to you about the Mother Nature's protection of the humanity's lifetime health, which is solely dependent on your lifetime consumption of mucilage. Why this mucilage is so critical is because the mucilage is what enables the body to use water from nature for the purpose of its proper hydration, and with this mucilage available plenty in your esophageal surface so that whenever you drink water it should wash some of it down and get it mixed in, and what happens here is proper hydration and this is how the Mother Nature turns the plain water from the nature into proper body fluid. But what happens if there was little or no mucilage available on the esophageal walls? I believe, in that case, the body rejects the water already introduced in the body starting an inflammatory action. As this process is repeated, I believe the inflammatory action is repeated and resulting aggravation works to build a chronic disease over time. I repeat. Plenty of mucilage on the walls of your esophagus from your daily consumption of mucilage rich foods will help ensure of your health year around, system-wide and naturally. And it includes your easy restful sleep night-after-night, proper musculature, bones and cartilage development and continued self-maintenance, all sexual as well as reproductive functions will be properly working. I dare say this is the core of the humanity's ever binding natural way of health program ensured by the Mother Nature, available to all individuals of humanity, regardless of racial differences, since thousands of years before the birth of modern medical science. This is an issue affecting us deeply as well as widely today. But as I see it the modern professionalized scientists are largely mum about this natural protection available to most everybody for pittance. I ask individuals go back to their conscious mind, get free of all the distractions and the noises around, concentrate on your true self interest and make a choice.

HERE ARE THE SIMPLE BASIC DIETARY CHOICES I MADE

— THE STUFF THAT IS "VISCOUS AND ELASTIC"
Choose any 3 of the items listed below, eaten with meals,
Twice a day every day, will Protect Your Lifetime Health:

//8 pcs raspberries// half slice avocado// 1 or 2 apricots, fresh or dried// 1/2 or 1 whole persimmon// 1 or 2 well ripen figs// 1 tsp to 1 Tbsp chia seeds necessarily pre-soaked in 1/2 to 1 full cup of water to avoid accidental intestinal blockage, and added to foods, soup or salad or simply cooked in the pot with water; long use history among Aztec Mexicans and the ancient Mayans in Middle America, who reputedly revered them as gift from gods// 1 tsp to 1 Tbsp flaxseeds (coarsely ground preferred or whole seeds pre-soaked in water); very long use history as medicine goes back 10,000 years, and a modern day functional food; the seeds come in two color, brown and golden; I like Bob's Golden Flaxseed Meal, 1-2 tbsp. Note: Golden Flaxseed is only produced in North Dakota is in limited supply and runs out quickly. The brown flaxseeds from the rest of the United States as well as Canada and Mexico are just as good.// 1 to 2 pcs okra fresh or frozen, sliced and added to foods// 1/4" to 1/2" slice Chinese yam or ma, with skin removed, edible fresh or cooked; the dried version of the same is a well known medicinal herb sanyao in the Traditional Eastern Medicine.// Seaweed called Dashima in Korean, also known as Sea Tangle, or Confu or Kunfu, usually soaked in water first, and then cooked with variable sea foods into a soup and then discard the Dashima seaweed; This traditional method popular in Japan and Korea reminds me of an American expression that goes "throwing away baby with bath water;" Therefore, I advocate a change, namely to chop up the seaweed and eat it, too as a valuable vegetable in the interest of protecting one's health from potential harms// Molokheia (Corchorus olitorius), also known as Egyptian spinach in the U.S.; This is the same plant that used to produce burlap bags, but its tender new leaves are popular as vegetable and healing herb in today's Egypt and several neighboring countries in the Middle East as well as unlikely places like Japan; Its long use history and reputation as healing herb goes back to pharaoh's ancient Egypt// Artichoke hearts sliced and frozen, a few slices with meal// Artichoke antipasto, 1 tsp to 1 Tbsp with meal// The use history of artichoke as a healing herb goes back to Romans and the Greek (Available at Trader Joe's)// Organic whole almond "fine ground meal' as produced and sold throughout Sprouts Farmers Markets in Northern California, where I live. In recent weeks I've come to love a mixture of this almond meal (2 Tbsp) and the golden flax meal given above (1 Tbsp) either added to my every meal or take a few tsp of the same mixture every time I use pomegranate juice preferred now diluted by 3-4 times of plain water. // Whole grains, some beans and various seaweeds can also be a valuable source of this essential nutrient in differing degrees. I use a few to several of the sources listed above all the time and I take no meals ever without them. I view the stuff that is "viscous and elastic" as my dietary health insurance personally, as well as the very nature's protection of humanity over the long evolutionary millions of years we came through until today. And I am very satisfied with it and deeply grateful for it. In our traditional diet I believe enough of it was contained in our daily food and that's how our body's health was more or less well protected. But as we entered the modern era and lost track of the traditional diet this nutrient, as it is often hidden from view, fell through the hole and we became deficient.

Chewy Vegetables Also Known As ROUGHAGES – My Mother loved them, and I love them, too.

My mother made a good impression on me chewing the hard to chew vegetables long and hard, saying, as if she needs to offer an apology, "You have to eat everything!" even on her false teeth since age 45 and until shortly before she passed away at age 96 in January 2018. I tend to credit her longevity to her lifelong dietary habit. And here are some chewy vegetables I love to eat: asparagus spears; fully grown purple chards with thick stems, golden beets, roots and tops; Korean radish tops, traditionally harvested when fully grown in early winter and dried under the north side eaves throughout the winter; and sweet potato leaves with stems peeled, traditionally poached and dried in the sun. I encourage you to find some roughages of your own choice and love them, too.

Although I am well aware of potential challenges some of my readers may face in this proposition, I am determined to show you how to get there. But you have to be willing to try my method, which is all natural and ordinary foods alone and expressly no medication except temporarily as may be needed, I mean you must love the Mother Nature's roughages yourself. For my method is based on my specialized experience only, which spanned over 6-7-8 years to complete, in addition to my earlier whole lifetime experience. It took much too long than I have imagined. Considering, however, that my problem of Yin Deficiency or Chronic Dehydration may have started in my early childhood and the age I started dietary study or experiment was fairly advanced at age 72, the resolution I have experienced was nothing less than extraordinary. I will further detail my experiences completely in this chapter. That's why I am willing to share my story with anybody who is willing to listen. If you are younger and healthier than I was the full benefits of the dietary measure should be realized much sooner. If you are in old age and with some chronic health issues you should expect a longer time frame for a full resolution. But you will get there eventually. I believe that is the nature's promise. The mucilage or soluble fiber attracts water strongly and can hold 1,000 times its dry measure of water. Therefore, expect to experience some strong dryness and itching on the skin as I described in earlier chapters, and sometimes it can be challenging. You can adjust the amount of mucilage you take from time to time to address your comfort level. Give your body time to work out all the details step by step. For me it took 7-8 years to reach complete freedom from my chronic disease that tortured me nearly 50 years and all other health troubles including from itching due to mucilage rich foods. For you it may be more or less depending your age and state of dehydration on your body. Be patient and continue with the recommended mucilage rich foods for life and your health will be protected. Medications may often present a short fix that may come with un-wanted side effects, sometimes worse than the previous affliction. I view most medications are unnecessary and often present distraction to our minds. It is imperative to keep our minds uncluttered and free so that we will stay independent and make proper judgment for our own best self-interest. I am saddened by stories of recent opioid epidemics and naturally weary of the expected introduction of marijuana. Be wary of short-term fixes! Take a long lifetime view and the right health option to support that view. Stand firm not be lured or stoop to trying narcotics even once, lest you may get trapped. It is often a trap. Once trapped, there's no easy way to get out. Health is the ultimate result of balance as I explained earlier. Seek for balance but not another medicine to distract your mind from the truth. In the long run, it's always the balance that determines your health. It's natural and easy. It may take time depending on where you are in your lifestyle. It's the smartest thing to try to live closer to or with Mother Nature.

This Is to Show How Nature Takes Care of the Humanity, Item by Item

In this section I will present some of the things I learned through my 6-7-8 years long use experiment with mucilage rich foods or the stuff that is "viscous and elastic" in a numbered sequence so that you the reader are informed of what kind of health benefits you can expect to obtain by using the same in your diet.

[1] FREE FLOW OF SALIVA IN THE MOUTH: Most people may take the saliva in their mouths for granted. But not everybody, for sure! Recently you may have heard in the news that some seniors complained of dry mouth with lack of saliva. Doctors are usually quick to attach a Greek nomenclature to the affliction but often unable to help relieve this condition. I once experienced this condition briefly, but my saliva flow was fully restored shortly after I started on my mucilage rich foods. I dare say simply, this is how Mother Nature works! The secret of the nature's wonder in keeping us alive and kicking is in the fact of proper hydration accomplished by the combination of water with mucilage in the esophagus as I explained earlier. It is the cornerstone of natural healing. Please make sure you understand this point correctly. To make sure whenever you drink water it shall properly hydrate you, you must have enough of mucilage in your esophagus by your habitual consumption of mucilage rich foods or soluble fiber all the time. You just make sure this requirement properly handled all the time, then most everything else will be done properly by your body *NATURALLY.*

[2] SLEEPING IS MADE EASY AND FULLY RELAXING NIGHT AFTER NIGHT: And ditto on my day naps every day. I knew that the Eastern Medicine teaches us that the Yin helps sleeping and in the earliest days of starting my food experiment in the year 2012 I slept soundly night after night. The difference was so stark and unmistakable because I have been a long chronically late and shallow sleeper. In earlier years, it had been my long habit to stay up late into the small hours most every night. But not anymore! I fall asleep effortlessly soon after I tucked myself into bed. Traditionally older people have been considered having sleeping problems because they tended to get dehydrated in Yin. But now with this mucilage rich, or Yin rich foods eaten everyday your Yin is fully supplied and as its result you can fall asleep soundly without any struggle. The enigma of sleeplessness is hereby finally solved! Come, all sleepless folks, try these mucilage rich foods and say, "No more insomnia!" I dare say simply, this is how Mother Nature works for ages!

[3] SEXUAL INTERCOURSE IS THE FIRST NATURAL STEP IN REPRODUCTION. TO MAKE THIS SUCCESSFUL AN ERECTION IS A NECESSARY PRE-CONDITION SINE QUA NON. Suffice it to say that this was one of my first three extraordinary impressions I experienced soon after starting mucilage rich, or Yin rich foods, probably within a month or two. Another health-related enigma of our time, the so-called erectile dysfunction hereby collapses. "No more erectile dysfunction, and for the woman, no more vaginal dryness, is the logical conclusion – as long as you consume enough of mucilage rich food every day!" I dare say simply, this is how Mother Nature works! This benefit is extended further to dramatically beautifying muscle and skin tones of the both of the sexes and possibly adding another dimension to enhancing intimacies.

[4] BY THE SAME TOKEN, THE NATURE'S PROTECTION SHOULD, AND DOES APPLY EQUALLY TO THE BODY OF WOMAN AS FAR AS REPRODUCTION IS CONCERNED FROM CONCEPTION THROUGH SUCCESSFUL DELIVERY OF A

HEALTHY BABY AND AS THE SUBSEQUENT BREAST-FEEDING LASTS, THE INTEGRITY OF WHICH IS ESSENTIAL TO SUCCESSFUL REPRODUCTION. THIS IS MY INFERENTIAL CONCLUSION. Therefore, I believe the regular consumption of mucilage rich, Yin Essence rich, or soluble fiber rich foods should protect woman's body so that these reproductive processes routinely and successfully conducted most every time as have been historically. In recent media reports I hear that woman's reproductive problems may have vastly increased. But our society has changed so that there are few people around them who are aware and ask questions about their nutrition due to erosion of credibility on the traditional diet. I believe most reproductive anomalies should be tied to the lack of adequate nutrition of soluble fiber. Simply, the nature's promise is unable to get implemented without this nutrition. Please be aware that due to the complexity of woman's reproductive organs, you may need a substantial lead time before the Mother Nature's protection starts kicking in after you started on this nutrient.

[5] SOLUBLE FIBER IS RESPONSIBLE FOR MANY ESSENTIAL FUNCTIONS IN PROTECTING HEALTH OF MEN AND WOMEN AS WELL AS CHILDREN AND SENIORS. MANY CHILDREN CATCH COLD OR OTHERWISE MISS THEIR SCHOOL DAYS AND WORKERS THEIR WORKDAYS. OLDER WOMEN OFTEN SUFFER FROM PERIMENOPAUSAL DISHARMONIES AND/OR URINARY DISORDERS, AND SOME EXPERIENCE VAGINAL DRYNESS. MOST OF THESE CAN BE ELIMINATED OR AT LEAST VASTLY REDUCED, IN MY OPINION, IF THEY USED ENOUGH OF SOLUBLE FIBER NURITION. BUT BE AWARE THAT YOU MAY NEED QUITE A LONG LEAD TIME BEFORE THE NATURE'S PROTECTION STARTS KICKING IN ONCE YOU STARTED MY RECOMMENDED DIET.

MY EARLIER NON-COMPLIANCE THROUGH MY YOUNGER YEARS OF MOTHER NATURE'S RULES HAD TO BE COMPENSATED FIRST BEFORE ANY FURTHER HEALING COULD TAKE PLACE. IT TOOK ME UPTO 6-7-8 YEARS TO SATISFY THE NATURE'S REQUIREMENT.

Let me explain a few loaded phrases I used above before starting my discussion on them. According to my understanding gained through my 6-7-8 years long and still going on mucilage rich, or Yin rich food consumption study, during the earlier period of my life before I started this study in March 2012 my body's constitution was marred (1) by lack of, or insufficiency of, my body's essential nutrients, chiefly the mucilage, or Yin Essence, or soluble fiber, (2) which hampered my body's proper hydration, (3) which caused over time a condition that I would call *The Chronic Dehydration Syndrome,* which harbored several diseases, (4) the chief among them was the sinus problem – unlimited source of unbearable miseries <u>involving the four of my five sense organs:</u> (Please read correction below.) My nose got stopped up and I couldn't breathe; my eyes were wet and constantly itching; my hearing and smelling were mostly completely blocked. These symptoms I suffered from in the worst possible period of my life while I started working first out of my graduate school in the U.S. and as a fresh immigrant, braving the harsh winter in Chicago. One day even my marriage ended. Those painful years are well passed now.

(Correction: My Chronic Dehydration affected all five of my five sense organs including my skin. Earlier I was mistakenly thought the black spots on top of my left shoulder and the several dark spots on both sides of my face on and around zygomatic arch, might have been result of sunburn, but I realized later that was a gross mistake. Now I know better: they are all direct results of my nearly 50 years-long sinus infection and the associated pathologies. If I were a woman, these dark spots especially those on the face would have been a serious issue. But I ignored them for years. In a physical exam 2 years ago just after moving into Los Gatos in the Northern California, the doctor noticed the dark spot on my left shoulder. It looked so bad that she wanted it checked out in case of any malignancy. It turned out okay, and soon in April 2020 we moved down to San Clemente in Orange County. I am glad I have found a simple but effective herbal tea to help restore the natural skin color as well as improve my complexion.

WHAT IS "THE PRIMARY INFLAMMATION"?

I now recall having read an article titled "The Primary Inflammation" on the Internet a few years ago, which I find since apparently been withdrawn. But I remember a few points of what the article said that when a chronic disease was associated with the Primary Inflammation it becomes incurable and the cause of the Primary Inflammation is unknown. I recall this mysterious "Primary Inflammation" in relation to what I termed "The Chronic Dehydration Syndrome" above. Now I wonder aloud if what this Primary Inflammation referred to was identical to my own term. I strongly suspect it is the very same thing. My Chronic Dehydration Syndrome was resistant to my healing efforts, but it eventually collapsed after 6-7-8 years continued effort consuming mucilage rich foods. Now I have proved what was previously thought incurable was effectively cured by my own dietary method without any drugs. But I suppose it still remains medically incurable. Besides I believe there is no way to circumvent the need of proper hydration otherwise and that's why the so-called Primary Inflammation was deemed incurable. But I say my self-treatment was done successfully by paying attention to the nature's rules – which ultimately are bogged down to proper hydration and restoring the damages wrought by repeated failures of proper hydration in previous years. **I strongly believe that the same experiment I ran over 6-7-8 years is completely replicable personally to whoever is willing to go through the same process in a number of years, which will be ultimately determined by his/her body's dehydration status. The final result is expected to be a complete healing free from all diseases on the person.** I believe the so called "Primary Inflammation" was incurable due to the fact that no proper and effective hydration was allowed to happen under the circumstances. But once a proper and effective hydration is allowed to happen the way I explain, the condition is likely to crumble from its impeccable perch eventually. A few such examples follow:

[6] DISEASE DUE TO CHRONIC DEHYDRATION #1: CHRONIC SINUS PROBLEM ALONG WITH THE ASSOCIATED MULTIPLE SENSE ORGAN PATHOLOGIES: This was a serious disease that tortured and ruined my life for decades. When I got determined to heal myself by natural means only, I got lucky to be able to defuse it naturally just like a fairy tale. The ease of it was so remarkable that I couldn't believe it, except that it took 6-7-8 long years for me to complete it in my body. Here is everything that I did, and what happened as a result:

A) Mucilage rich, Yin rich, or soluble fiber rich foods as I described above, used twice everyday as part of the meals, started in March 2012, was the main measure of my self-treatment providing proper hydration as well as correcting previous years of failed hydration caused chronic pathologies due to dehydration, and as I describe in the next item [5] A) soon after a memorable event occurred in May 2018 my hearing blockage was completely disappeared. What I call a memorable event marked the completion of the proper rehydration of all the cells and tissues of my digestive tract as I understand it, and the final and complete healing of my chronic sinus problem was in the offing. And I am still continuing my diet as of 7/15/2018. Of course, I am still continuing my mucilage and committed to do so as long as I may live as my lifetime health plan as of today, Tuesday, April 28, 2020.

B) My seemingly magic potion consisting of 1/3 cup Lakewood Organic Pure Pomegranate Juice, 1/3 cup Blue Diamond Almonds, Unsweetened Original Almond Breeze almond milk, and 1/3 cup water added to dilute and stirred up to get the contents evenly mixed (best tasting if poured in this order) and drunk immediately after meals; and repeat the same after each time waking up from bed and/or naps. As of now 7/15/2018, fully 2 years and 3 months, I feel I am free from my sinus problem and may no longer need this drink because I feel that the healing action back into the chronic dehydration may have reached far enough. But I got used to it since March 2016 and I like it. The mix makes a well-balanced and pleasing drink, and I may continue to use it in lieu of water. I still love and continue the drink after each meal only. 8/21/18. I reaffirm the usefulness of this mixed drink perhaps as a digestive aid or something hard for me to point out, and I am firmly in favor of using this drink indefinitely in the future. 11/03/18. Shortly thereafter as of 12/17/18, however, I am mulling over replacing this once my favorite drink by 2 heaping tsp of almond meal and 1/3 cup of Apple Mango Nectar from France, eat it like a loose porridge with a spoon and then rinse the bowl with 1/3 cup of water and drink it, each time after meal and after getting up out of bed, total 4 times daily. I eventually dropped almond drink outright, and instead I adopted whole organic almond kernels more liberally with the understanding that they apparently are very helpful to my digestive process toward health. I have started to use whole almond kernels in two ways. One of the ways, I take 24 kernels of whole almonds (about 1 oz.) and roast them 4-5 minutes in a small pan, chew the half of them right after the meal with a drink of 1/3 cup of pomegranate juice diluted by an equal measure of water. I save the other half of the roasted almond kernels and use them the same way after I wake up from the night sleep or from a daily nap. And I also take another 24 kernels of whole almonds, soak 24 hours and add them to my day time pot just once a day, which I never repeated and dropped out completely because I found the resulting cooked almond skins were found too tough to chew. Lately, I got attracted by the convenience of ready to use almond tortilla sheets. I wish these were organic, but I find the convenience hard to beat and tend to use the most. And I consider almond and the pomegranate juice as a pair to go together. I like them both that way.

C) Obviously, I ate other items of foods in my meals, relatively simple and largely fixed but a pretty good variety in my opinion. a) Grains and beans: I use only coarsely milled grains to retain as much fiber as possible such as long grain red wild rice, red sorghum, and "rat eye" small black beans, soaked 24 hours and cooked in electrical rice cooker on mixed grains mode, transferred to a plastic container, cooled off and stored in the refrigerator, used 2-3 Tbsp in each of my twice daily meals to last 5-7 days, then the same process has to be repeated; Partly due to my laziness in repeating this cumbersome chore and partly due to the digestive sluggishness I experience I tend to omit this entirely recently, but within a couple of weeks I decided that I would rather continue to use some amount of my mixed grains and beans in my daily meals. In spite of what I said above, I look forward to phasing out my consumption of whole grain rice, sorghum and beans due to digestive difficulty as well as their required extra chore of preparation taxing on my increasingly lazy body as I get older and the increased use of whole almonds turns out to supplant them pretty well as I expect so. b) A sizzling hot pot twice daily, at noon and at midnight: As I get older, I tend to refrain from red meat and prefer fish and plant foods; I used to enjoy sardines and herrings from Korean coastal seas and look for something similar in Northern California, where I now live. I try smart with whatever I find I like every time I shop. It's a struggle, often ending up with a mixed bag of small things including shellfishes because I generally look for the smaller ones for less contamination. And this is how I arrange my pot: I take $1/8^{th}$ vertical slice of a large golden beet root and further slice it into two equal slices and arrange them to face each other vertically about 1-2 inches apart. (And I used to add small slices of Trader Joe's Twin Pack Organic Sprouted Tofu, which yields 8 servings for me. I used this for the purpose of preventing occasional nasal sniffles. I believe this condition has been largely cleared by the power of proper hydration having reached to the bottom of my nasal cavities, and therefore I discontinue its use as of 7/31/18.

D) And subsequently in a few days I decided to reduce the golden beet root down to a 1/8 slice and a leafy stem of red chard as of 8/4/18.) And then I pour 12 hour-presoaked small pieces of Dashima in 1/2 cup of water at the center of the pot and between the facing twin slices of golden beet root. And then at the center on top of Dashima I drop 4 pcs of asparagus spears. I may also throw in a few slices of frozen artichoke bulb. Lately, I prefer to use a thin slice of ma, instead. And I place whatever fish, half thereof, or fishes on top of Dashima and asparagus spears. The fish is the main source of my protein and since I am well experienced in the amino acids lysine over arginine imbalances I am careful to get enough lysine but not too much protein, which may lead to gaining weight, and eventually toward inflammation, for my ultimate goal is complete freedom from disease and pain by maintaining any potential inflammation down to zero, while getting enough nutrition for my healthy living. Once I've got a one kilo package of tiny frozen squids and used 5 of them with some dried strips of Pollack, and I found them very satisfying. If I had some frozen peeled baby shrimps and/or small shelled shellfish I would throw a bunch of them, but I ran out of them this week. I've trialed various fishes, and eventually last week when I found at the Trader Joe's that they have smaller and more or less uniform serving sized frozen sockeye salmon slices in stock and decided to make that my choice of fish from now on. 8/14/18. Shortly thereafter I quit sockeye salmon entirely and its stead I used small bunches of smaller and non-fatty sea foods such as small shrimps, baby clams, and mussels to see if these will help sufficiently with my need of daily protein. So far it turned out surprisingly well that I am pleased that I got rid of the fatty salmon and as a result my waistline was given a little breathing slack. As I wrote in the previous chapter, I value cacao nibs highly as a heart healthy natural food and I add 1 level Tbsp of it to every pot of my meal. The rest of the ingredients into my sizzling pot of meal are my usual favorite vegetables such as either Kabocha or butternut squash pcs, purple sweet potato pcs, if available, or Korean/Japanese sweet potato pcs., a large coarse chard leaf with purple stem chopped and used as cover (This week I ran out of it.) I also add 8pcs of Ginko nuts as tonic to my lungs because I had history of asthma. Occasionally I add some of my home grown large tasty beans known as scarlet emperor. With beautiful red flours and showy vines this plant is often favored as an ornamental. I value it as an attractive edible landscaping plant in my small shady backyard. On top I scatter chopped red jalapeno pepper. This week I ran out of it and substituted a green jalapeno from my backyard. I eventually gave up on hot peppers entirely on 8/21/18. My older body can't stand it anymore. I still craved some spice and also had an issue with flatulence because of my high fiber mixed grains and beans. I got an idea, which I hoped might help solve both of these problems. So I went to an Indian grocery and bought small (200g each) packages of turmeric powder, kasmiri chili powder and crushed fenugreek seeds. I tried 1/4 tsp each sprinkled over my pot. The spice failed even registering on my tongue. Then I doubled it, which gave a mild taste and a great reduction of flatulence. I think I'll keep it that way. But later I reduced the herbs back to 1/4 tsp each and I mean to keep it there indefinitely. With 1 and 3/4 cups of water, I sizzle it for the first 10 minutes at the maximum heat, 5 minutes at 1/2 heat and finish it with 5 minutes at low heat, [or with 2 full cups of water, after the first 10 minutes reduce heat by 1/2 and continue

10 minutes and stop. In this scenario make sure that you have enough water to go through all the way.] Thus, cooking is done in 20 minutes. And then a drizzle of perilla seed oil, rich in omega 3 fatty acids and then a few quick squirts of coconut vinegar over it. No salt added. I recently quit soy sauce, too. I found the sea foods without salt added are good enough. That's about it. Twice a day, at noon and at midnight. (Note: Both golden beet and chard are botanically known as Beta vulgaris and both are highly anti-inflammatory. And that's why I choose them. Beet root is quite sweet and that's why I use a small fraction of it.) 8/1/18. I also have a habit of munching on some fruit of various kinds as an appetizer and desert. A 1/2 slice of avocado is one of my favorites. I've found coarsely ground golden flax seeds and added them to my hot pot, alternately with chia seeds, replacing avocado. 11/03/18.

E) Bamboo Shoots were one of my first choices of foods I selected for the purpose of fighting my chronic sinus problem. At first I used a good slice of it as one of the regular ingredients for my hot pot, and had a small slice also as a snack along with a small slice of sprouted tofu every time I had a drink of my so called magic potion as referenced above on item B), that is, immediately after every meal as well as immediately after waking up from bed or from naps for a few years. Besides, during the first few months I felt I had to repeat the bamboo, tofu and drink routine every time I woke up in the night, sometimes more than once a night, I got sick and tired of these extra chores I felt I had to perform and gradually reduced to just once a night. Then in January 2018 my Old Mother passed away, so I left all these chores behind and flew to Korea to attend her funeral in Korea. When returned back home the next month I practically 'forgot' everything about the bamboo shoots, but just kept steady with all the details of the above three A), B), and C) as described. As luck would have it, however, my health went largely unaffected because by the time my body's progressing deep tissue healing must have reached, in my understanding, nearly far enough correcting the damages caused by the dehydration due to the previous long history of hydration failure. The only inconvenient side effect of discontinuing the bamboo shoots was occasional sniffles. I often had to resort to eating a slice of the sprouted tofu, which was largely effective. By the end of July 2018, the sniffles have largely gone. It's simply exhilarating! Sorry, I realize now it was not true. My once a chronic disease, that is, sinus condition has been completely uprooted and gone by my mucilage rich diet. But I still have some sniffles usually after getting up from bed or a nap and I have to blow my nose a few to several times. I think this is due to the fact that I had allowed a Virginia ENT to puncture my left eardrum 5 years ago for drainage purposes and I am left wondering if it can be possibly undone. My guess is probably not, so I must endure it as long as I would. 2/19/19.

But later throughout March 2019 I experienced vastly increased clear nasal mucous. A bit earlier when my son was here, I loved walking with his dog Singy and I ran into trouble hitting my head against an electrical pole hard and I heard the "crack" on my forehead and I collapsed on the ground there. I was immediately taken to an urgent care place and had an X-ray scan and was told that it showed that there was "a significant inflammation in my sinuses", so I eventually agreed with my daughter to see an ENT doctor. (My daughter had taken me to see a local ENT on Thu. May 2, 2019, who found a polyp in my right-side nose and recommended a nasal spray to let it shrink away. When I declined to use the spray saying that it was on the way of healing and may soon disappear, the doctor offered to see me again to check on it in 6 months. This was what my daughter old me when I asked her about it on Sat., May 19, 2019.)

[7] DISEASE DUE TO CHRONIC DEHYDRATION #2: CHRONIC CONSTIPATION AND THE EVENTUAL PROPER CELLULAR RE-HYDRATION OF MY ENTIRE DIGESTIVE TRACT

A) I was greatly surprised that while I was continuously taking mucilage rich, Yin Essence rich, or soluble fiber rich foods over 6 years faithfully twice every day, when a memorable event occurred to me some time in May 2018 that made me convinced that my body's progressing and slowly advancing proper hydration, which may have started in my mouth, the proximal opening of my body's digestive tract, and apparently progressed cell by cell, tissue by tissue, taking over 6 years of time in doing so, must have finally reached and/or penetrated the tissues of the distal end of the same digestive tract, thus completing what I consider to be "the Proper Cellular Hydration" of the entire digestive tract of my body. A few months earlier during my trip to Korea and back most of my sense organs were working relatively comfortable except my ears, which were hard of hearing to some degree, which must have annoyed and worried my son. When we reached San Jose railroad station, where he was to take a train for Southern California, and I was to take a cab home nearby, he lectured on me in a manner as if he were a parent of me and I were his child. I was so ashamed and protested screaming loudly. The station was deserted and there was no one around us. I have never made good money in my life and when I reached retirement age, I had little savings. I was earlier concerned about dementia as a side effect of taking the sinus medication, and as soon as I realized that I immediately discontinued the medication. During the Korea trip I happened to mention to my son about that. I have been taken in with my daughter and her family and if there were any unusual expenses such as medical my son was expected to chip in. I originally planned to continue my acupuncture practice to my age 100 but it didn't work out that way and fell through the hole. Then I turned my mind back to my penchant dream that I wanted to make really a significant contribution to people's health in my lifetime somehow. The one dream slipped out of my hand but I'm going to see through this one. My hearing was probably blocked one last time during and immediately after the Korean trip. My hearing as of now 12/22/2019, is free from any blockages and completely restored. A happy ending!!!

After the memorable event in May 2018, I mentioned above, things moved rather quickly, I mean the healing of my body that I have been so patiently waiting for all those years. I felt as if the very root of constipation as well as the seat of my body's chronic dehydration syndrome that was entrenched there for decades was finally effectively uprooted and ejected out of my body. I felt so light as if I could walk freely. Now that the Spleen, which I understand to be equivalent to the digestive tract, has been restored, it starts to take care of my limbs, as the Eastern Medicine says, I thought. But the flimsy euphoria lasted only for a day or two. Rightly thereafter, my right leg felt dangling at each of the three joints, namely, at hip, knee and ankle as if indicating that all the cartilage has been completely worn out. Then quickly again it changed to a 'wet and heavy' feeling, becoming increasingly heavier as days went on. I do not know but I guess that my body is going to regenerate my cartilage and restore my joints like new, sort of. I am looking forward to seeing that materialize. I tend to believe that what I called the flimsy euphoria was a flash card by which my body showed me its plan and how it is going to be like when it is completed. The next month the progressing proper rehydration has apparently reached the tissues in my head and cleared my hearing completely – no more obstruction, or any hard of hearing! More on my right leg, later.

[8] DISEASE DUE TO CHRONIC DEHYDRATION #3: DEMENTIA:

Within a few months my ears were completely clear of any blockages, and I was eager to see any signs that would improve my memory because the Eastern Medicine says the Yin protects the memory. Since my brain and the tissues holding the memory are within relatively a close proximity in the head from the ears and nasal cavities, where I am assured that the progression of proper hydration, according to my theory, must have reached by now I was eagerly looking forward to seeing some signs of my memory improving. It did not help. At this point of time 12/22/19, memory recall is possible but has become vastly slow. When my son visited me in April, I told him I was ahead of him, meaning that I was already aware of the issues of my memory and trying to prevent any catastrophic event as long as I live. At least that is my goal at this time. Occasionally I catch myself letting things slip by, but I am still positive about my memory holding on so that I can manage my life as I have been doing so far.

But I am well aware that my effort to maintain my memory may be a struggle or a fight. Here is my strategy on how to do it to maintain an upper hand to the end, and hopefully the recovered proper hydration may come to the aid in preserving my memory. My analysis so far tells me that there is another step before dementia steps in and that is a sort of attention deficit. Normally I used to do things in a flowing continuity, but now it happens sometimes like, for example, when I was working at the kitchen I needed something from my room so immediately my feet take me to the room but when I reached the room I forgot what it was that I wanted. To prevent this kind of situation from happening again, I want to say aloud like "I want to get my water bottle," or something like that. Having a thought briefly fails to stay in my mind and I fail to recollect it. So from now on I plan to make sure each moment of thought is registered in my mind, and in that case I have no trouble so far in recalling it. Make sure to register your thought in your mind. That's my strategy fighting not to fall unto the slippery slope that may lead to dementia. Conscious living, that is. I have always valued maintaining my conscious mind. A slow deliberate step after step…

CHEWING MAINTAINS HIPPOCAMPUS-DEPENDENT COGNITIVE FUNCTION

Huayue Chen, Mitsuo Iinuma, [….], and Kin-Ya Kubo

ABSTRACT Mastication (chewing) is important not only for food intake, but also for preserving and promoting the general health. Recent studies have showed that mastication helps to maintain cognitive functions in the hippocampus, a central nervous system region vital for special memory and learning. The purpose of this paper is to review the recent progress of association between mastication and the hippocampus-dependent cognitive function. There are multiple neural circuits connecting the masticatory organs and the hippocampus. Both animal and human studies indicated that cognitive functioning is influenced by mastication. Masticatory dysfunction is associated with hippocampal morphological impairments and the hippocampus-dependent spatial memory deficits, especially in elderly. Mastication is an effective behavior for maintaining the hippocampus-dependent cognitive function in older people. We also discussed several possible mechanisms involved in the interaction between mastication and the hippocampal neurogenesis and the future directions for this unique fascinating research.

Keywords: Cognition, Hippocampus, Mastication

https://www.ncbi.nlm.nih.gov>articles

I've made some light flavored kimchi with long dakuan type radish roots and tops and found them pleasantly hard to chew and yet eventually chewable!!! And I found it helping clear up some fuzzy stuff in my head immediately. The experience is positively enlivening, and I want to go further. I will get some chewy dried stuff like squid and enjoy extra 15-30-45 min. chewing them as snack. I bought some dried squids and chew them while I prepare my meals twice a day. Yum!!! After a few to several weeks as of 12/17/2018 I already feel a lot better. I feel I am holding myself on for the time being. But I eventually dropped this idea of chewing dried squids due to its side effect, which is, producing an excess of saliva, which washed out my gummy surfaces and apparently promoting inflammation when sugary substances from my deserts impacted my gummy surfaces and causing pain as of 1/22/2019. I can still eat my radish kimchi but tend to neglect it lately. Yes, I'm still committed to chewable foods of different kinds like roasted whole almond kernels and some chewy small fishes such as squids, octopuses' slices, mussel, cuttlefish, clams, etc. I keep on going committed to protecting my memory as a functioning self-help individual as long as I can. So far I'm doing well. 2/19/2019.

I am going to share one of my recent food searching stories with you. In recent years I liked almond milk and pomegranate juice, which led me to get eventually interested in whole almonds rather than just drinking the blanched almond milk. I thought this was just a progression of my natural interest for I always considered myself basically a naturalist and what is the natural is the best food for me. So, when I sought to add more almonds to my food I looked around and bought some almond flour tortillas but my basic mode of basically two pots roasts a day, making everything conform with this style eventually and therefore supplemented them with everything else that was lacking, such as Organic Almond Meal by Sprouts Farmers Market. Eventually I progressed to having a large bowl of salad for my daytime meal, and a cooked pot as usual only for my nighttime meal.

[9] DISEASE DUE TO CHRONIC DEHYDRATION #4: MY RIGHT LEG:

I mentioned about an auto accident in 1995, in which I had my left leg tibia broken. It was treated in cast and then got healed after weeks of physical therapy and I soon joined a hiking group. During the next 10 years or so I became one of the most enthusiastic members of the group and forgot all about the injury I sustained earlier. Then about 10 years later in 2014 when I visited my son in Utah, we had a hike and I found I constantly lagged behind and could not keep up with him and his children. I wondered aloud what my problem was. In my earlier hiking group, there were a few older hikers in their 70's and even 80's. They walked just as well as the rest of us. I had assumed when I came of their ages I would walk just as well as they did. What was wrong with me? I was left perplexed. When I moved to Northern California in 2016, I happened to live right next to a county park and a long streamside trail, an ideal place for someone who loves hiking like me. But the physical condition I was in was not apparently ideal. It became increasingly difficult to walk in the next couple of years, so I had an X-ray taken to find out why. The results described in my doctor's letter were unremarkable and commented saying "Good for your age." But the condition I have been experiencing is anything but good. Soon after I arrived here in Northern California my buttocks felt heavy. And a year earlier when I hiked with my son and his children I lagged and was unable to keep up with them. I failed to understand what was happening to my body. It has become clear to me now that those were the early harbingers alerting me of what was coming in my right leg. In the last few months, I cut back walking sharply. Now I hardly go out of the door except on weekly shopping trips. Now I even neglect watering my backyard garden plants and let them shrivel up and die. My body is so lazy and tired that I couldn't care any longer. 8/25/18. Probably 6-12 months ago, I felt all three of my right leg joints were dangling briefly for a week or so, and then for a day or two it seemed well connected if it were flimsy and I felt I could walk freely just like a dream-like sensation. My body may have showed this to me like a flash card premonition, I surmised later. After that brief moment of Shangri-La my right leg turned heavy and with a distinctively wet sensation, as if dripping wet, but just in my sensation alone. Several months later I don't have the wet sensation any longer. For several weeks now I have managed taking a daily walking, what I termed a vigorous walking with fairly quick and long strides circling the large tri-angular block along Blossom Hill Road/ Los Gatos Blvd/ Robert Road in front of the middle school, two full rounds in 55 minutes from leaving my room and returning back. The walking is increasingly difficult now. If my leg is going through a healing process, which I believed in the beginning, I still stand by my belief but getting tired of a long wait. As of now 12/17/18 I barely make one round daily and have to wonder what's ahead of me. **What I thought a small Big Toe Mishap 20+years ago, now at age 79 seems to be** causing a permanent disability in walking is an undeniable mystery illness. It is so complex in symptoms and difficult to describe. A small rubber insert given by the doctors does not seem to correct anything but make it barely bearable: As of 12/22/19.

[10] SOME LITTLE BUT OBNOXIOUS NUISANCES ON MY BODY

A) Dandruff! Oh! I hated it! Through my entire life! Starting in my middle school years when my social self-image was budding! Never disappeared completely no matter what I did! Finally rendered rarefied or non-existent in my twilight years and very recently! 8/24/18. My dandruff is gone and completely clear now 12/17/18. Maybe I was wrong. It's scarce but still hanging around some, and when I forgot to wash my hair and the next evening, I got itch and had some dandruff still there. The daily maintenance I have been doing is essential to keep it low and out of trouble, 1/30/19. This now convinces me that I was actually have been lacking proper hydration for a long time even into my youth and probably even later.

B) So called athlete's foot fungal disease, and another one I love to hate. It can be kept hidden under the socks and I ignored it for long. My right big toe apparently got injured, and when I crawled as a baby I cried because of pain, my mom told me. The injury apparently has never healed and eventually my big toenail got infected presenting a thick ugly unruly thing I learned to hate. Recently I visited a podiatrist in hope that the infected nail may be pulled out so that a new nail free from infection may grow. I am given up on that chance now and satisfied in maintenance care that I dutifully administer every night after bath. 8/24/18. I apply FUNGI NAIL dutifully every night. That takes care of it and I continue to comply with it. I can't think of any natural way to defeat this infection. And in the recent several months the same right big toe was stiff, numb and hurting but I was ignoring it. This was the big toe that was injured about 10 years ago when I was hiking in North Carolina on November first with the first snow flurries that year. I finished my intended hiking that day nonetheless and eventually found the big toe twitched a bit to the right pushing the other toes further sideways. I ignored it for 10 years and why is it hurting now? I know this is because my body's natural self-healing due to my continued use of mucilage rich foods must have finally reached my big toe. I know because I have had a similar experience a few years ago on my left leg after it was injured two decades ago. I believe this was the delayed healing due to the failure of hydration for two decades and as the proper hydration was finally accomplished the true healing has started taking place. It's going on now and it will be done when it runs its course. I just have to wait it out. With this I have a new hope now that I may be able to defeat my lifetime big toenail infection that may have started when I was a crawling baby. I'll watch and report to you. 1/30/18. [Unfinished]

C) Itchy little bumps appeared on the medial side of my both wrists in my 30's or 40's. I never knew why but they have completely disappeared only on recent months leaving no trace. Were they caused by dehydration? Possibly, but I do not know for sure. Just glad to be ridden of! 8/24/18. They are completely gone and clear now 12/17/18.

D) Itchy Dark ominous looking quarter-sized sunburn spot on top of my left shoulder raised concern of skin cancer. I took a skin biopsy, which showed a seborrheic keratosis. There was no atypia or malignancy, the test report said. 09/09/2016. Healed well and never reappeared 12/17/18. I used to think this was caused by sunburn, but now it appears more likely an extended aftermath of my sinus/ear infection. The next item E) ditto in this regard.

E) Dark sunburn spots on both sides of my face at or around zygomatic arch: could have been a serious matter if I were a woman. But I didn't care much and don't even remember when they started to appear. I do remember they used to be much larger, the size of a nickel, and in recent years got shrunk down to the size of a dime. Their sizes are getting smaller and smaller while the darkness is becoming lighter and lighter. I think their complete disappearance appears likely in a few more years. They are still there as of 12/17/18. I used to largely ignore them so far, and then recently as I was getting older, I wanted to see if I could make them smaller and get smaller as I go I stared smear a little almond oil every time right after taking bath. This I have done in the past several months and find them getting lighter in the color and smaller in sizes, so I have decided to continue it every night. 2/10/20.

F) This item is not about something new, but a reassessment on the above items both D) and E). Initially I thought they were caused by solar radiation, but now I say I was so naïve and ashamed of it. I have no doubt at all but now I am 100% sure that they were all the results of my now infamous sinus troubles. My left ear got infected even before I realized it.

Addendum: Some Small Lifesavers I Love

- This way I protect my lungs. Lungs need more than good nutrition: warmth and freedom from irritants that may be in the air. Normally food intake creates and increases the amount of heat body needs. As my body ages I get the impression that there may be a double whammy of aging effect that on the one hand my body's ability to produce heat on the set amount of food is on the decrease, and my body's interest in increased intake of food as well as the ability to process it also is on the decrease. So, if this is true, which I think so, my options left are putting on extra layers of clothing and a space heater. Fortunately, I live in the mild climate in Northern California, where freezing temperature is rare. I have an electrical space heater set at 70 degrees just in case the night temperature dips below zero and it rarely does. So, my main and favorite adjustment to help keep my lungs warm and secure is putting on extra clothing and I go quite a bit of distance in this regard. I see three steps of symptoms in which the lungs complain of being chilled: the mildest may be some nasal discharge or sniffles, the next step closer to a disease is sneezing, which is usually sudden, violent and often recurring, and the last is cough, which is already a form of disease. I read that quite a few of seniors die of pneumonia and I think this kind of personal self-care practice may help protect the individuals before being placed on the slippery slope toward pneumonia. This should show that personal self-care practices are really vital in protecting our health, a serious life-threatening disease usually does not happen overnight, and as long as we stay aware we can find a way to prevent them, and the Mother Nature is on our side with us just taking a simple nutrition. And we can easily put on another layer of clothing or two to keep warm. In these days in October and November I often don on a jacket even indoors, and when I sit at my desk, I usually drape an old shirt over my knees to keep them comfortable. And in the night, I wear double warm shirts in the bed and use an old jacket insert that is thick and warm to cover my chest and place an old woolen scarf across my shoulders and keep my arms out. Then I pull up the bedding to my sternum, or all the up to the chin depending on my comfort level. This arrangement gives me a bed that is just right, very comfortable every night. I enjoy deeply relaxing sleep night after night, thanks to my mucilage rich foods. I rarely kick or otherwise disturb my bed. I just slip in and slip out, every night, and ditto on my day naps every day. My bed is made once a week with fresh linens.

- I also want you to know about a special food to protect your lungs: ginko nuts. Gingko or Eunhaeng in Korean, meaning Silver Apricot, was never grown in farms in Korea when I lived there but picked up from wild stands in the late fall through early winter, often offered as nibbling snack by roadside food sellers or beer shops, often skewered in a toothpick and lightly roasted with a sprinkling of salt. There is a Korean saying that goes: "Even the Eunhaeng trees must stand face to face to bear fruit" about their sexual reproduction. This unique living fossil tree of prehistoric origin offers a special tonic to those of us who has deficiency of Lung Qi according to the Traditional Eastern Medicine. Since I have history of asthma and being short of breath, I thought I could benefit from eating this unusual food, now regularly stocked with Chinese imports in my local Korean food store. I continue eating this nut, 8 pcs per meal, twice a day, as one of my essential daily foods. Recently I checked on the Web and found a website saying an excessively large amount of ginko nuts may lead to an incurable toxicity, and another site recommending 10 nuts maximum and not to eat anymore. I have been eating 8pcs twice a day (or 16 pcs per day) of ginko nuts cooked in my food for a number of years and I haven't experienced any adverse effect whatsoever. My purpose of using this food in my daily fare is to prevent any chances of developing conditions that may lead to pneumonia later. But I would advise any interested potential users to proceed with due personal diligence and caution. It is my personal mantra that says, "a cough may be a step to catching cold and catching cold may be a step to pneumonia to a senior person, which may be a sure path to death. I also have a similar caution on fall while being a senior.

- Another special food to protect, hopefully, my memory, this time. Can lotus seeds be helpful in preserving memory function longer? I don't know it for sure, but I have been using them recently for several months and I tend to think so. In the Traditional Chinese/ or Oriental Medicine Yin is ultimately considered responsible for protecting memory. Earlier in this book, I explained how water drunk into the body can protect us against inflammation in the body by the help of fiber and water in the diet. I emphasized that without proper fiber in the diet, true hydration of the body cells cannot be obtained but necessarily inflammation is caused, which starts a disease, and over time a chronic disease materializes. This is my opinion at this time, and probably scientific community has not offered anything definitive on the process of hydration. Now I do not know but I tend to believe that lotus seeds may have a function in helping preserve water in the memory retaining brain cells. And I eat 6 pcs of soaked lotus seeds, either raw or cooked with foods twice every day. I believe this may be helpful in protecting my memory. I passed my 80th birthday a few months ago. 2/11/20, Ditto, I get more positive, 3/16/20.

- Almond Oil, organic, non-GMO, cool, expeller pressed, food grade only; relieved, and healed itching flea bites; reduced and healed measles rashes on my little daughter sooner than otherwise; my all-around skin emollient, antiseptic, anywhere on my body where I can reach, can't do without this essential personal treasure.

- For bath I have been long a reluctant user of all those abrasive chemicals found in soaps, shampoos and conditioners. I let them rest now. Instead, I quickly squeeze out a drop of my organic olive oil out of my small bottle oil dispenser under the hot bath water I have just turned on and adjust the water temperature to make it just right. The hot water lets the oil break up into tiny almost invisible particles and spread over more or less evenly. I walk in and sit in the warm water, rinse my face with a small cotton hand-towel. (Later I changed into hemp cloth towel and like it better.) Then I plunge full length in the water and relax a few minutes. Then I take a scratchy kind of bath towel (I utilize what Korean stores sell for rice cake steaming hemp cloth for this purpose.) and run over my entire body surface a couple of times. Then I kneel over the water and rinse my scalp and hair several times. That's about it – in about half an hour bathing is done. I used to struggle with persistent severe dandruff all my life and several skin rashes and boils here and there. All those got completely cleaned up in the wake of my over 8 years long use of mucilage rich foods. So, my simplified bath now leaves me good and refreshed every time. This way my skin is left moist, supple and not too dry or itchy as it used to be. The skin is the largest of my five sense organs, and as such specially organized for the role of protecting the whole body. As I said earlier again and again this important job is accomplished by the use of simple biotechnology of using the mucilage food. I am presenting a proof of what this particular nutrient can do for your skin. The use of almond oil in my bath is just putting the last touch of my self-care regime toward the well-being of my body and spirit.

- I am also using a dietary measure to prevent a catastrophic event such as heart-attacks or strokes, that is, one Tbsp each of organic raw cocoa nibs twice a day, either sprinkled over salad, or cooked with foods. May be an extra chore, but who knows. I'd rather stay protected than otherwise. That's a prevention minded person's logic.

- Wild dandelions self-planted appear here and there in the backyard. A palm sized tuft appears enticing to be tossed into the salad bowl. Several of them ended up in my salad bowl over a few weeks. The cooling weather in October into November has chilling effect in the new sprout and makes me realize I have to wait for the next spring, when I will be happy to oblige. (I have recently decided to clean out all dandelions or dandelion- look alike weeds, in the back yards. As my appetite decreases, I don't care about them as free salad source any longer. I pulled them all out. Now I'm posed to move to Southern Calif.)

- In the popular culture I notice a little sugar is added here and there quite often. This statement in itself is not an issue. But the culture it represents is a huge health threat, a real and practical issue that the whole world of the modern societies faces today struggling. A simple and real break to this huge problem can only come from a conscious mind of individuals like you and me, realizing that any excess calories are going to add to the inflammatory pressure eventually causing a disease. Most natural foods are good tasting without any added sugar. Once again, sugar increases inflammation, which incubates a disease. If you want to stay free from disease and pain you need to stay free from extra calories or sugar. Consider never buying sugar at all as a practical measure. This may be a fundamentally a most practical decision in the way of staying free from disease and pain. At this early stage a decision to prevent can be easily and effectively made. Later on, however, when a disease fully matured it could amount to a life and death issue on top of the huge monetary costs, which is what we really choose to end up with, although unconsciously so, because procrastination is often the game plan most of us are guilty of. We must wake up to this realization. Prevention pays. Limiting extra calories and sugar is the very fundamental step in prevention. And it's the only best option because it is the cheapest as well as the easiest and the most effective.

- My reluctant radish kimchi making delivers huge health dividends overnight and got my slowed kimchi making interest rekindled by mainly and effectively helping reduce memory loss pressure. I also bought some dry squids, which are quite chewy. I like to chew a small piece while preparing for my meal. The practice brings out saliva and may help digest my meal when ready. Anyway, I find these extra chewing practices have turned out to be uniquely responsible for stopping my once worrisome memory loss pressure and stabilized the situation into an acceptable manner It feels like almost a 'miraculous' feat. I would highly recommend any of my fellow senior readers to consider this approach. My radish kimchi making still continuing as of 6/6/20.

- Sprouted Tofu Helps Reduce Flatulence. "It is well known that consumption of pulses leads to flatulence. Inclusion of legumes in the diet at levels that provide 20-25 percent of total calories results in a manifold rise in the amount of gas produced in the intestines. Studies in humans fed different pulses have shown that chickpea is more gas-forming than other pulses. One of the factors associated with flatulence is the high concentration in pulses of certain oligosaccharides of the raffinose family. Because of the absence of suitable digestive enzymes these sugars are not utilized by man. The unabsorbed sugars are acted upon by the micro-flora of the large intestine resulting in gas production. Studies on common pulses like the chickpea, green gram, black gram, and red gram have indicated a continuous fall on oligo-sugar content on germination. In grains germinated for twenty-four hours the oligo-sugar levels are at 50 percent of their initial value, and by 48-72 hours at less than 25-15 percent. These observations suggest that sprouted pulses are likely to be less flatus-producing. Quoted from *Germination and malting* posted on archive.unu.edu of U.N. University, India, accessed Jan. 3, 2016.

- A small bamboo back-scratcher, nicknamed as a "dutiful child's hand," but I think this is better than being scratched by fingernails including even those of a dutiful child. Scratching by fingernails can add to the inflammatory pressure that may already be present, but the bamboo, which is known to have cooling energy in the Traditional Eastern Medicine, may really offer help to reduce itching. I firmly believe so and that's why I always keep a bamboo back-scratcher close to me as a little lifesaver.

- As I get tired and lazy, I cut back most of cooking and tend to make uncooked meals or salads some of the times nowadays. For a snack, I place a half piece of flat persimmon/sliced, an apricot/sliced and a few red raspberries, blackberries and/or blueberries in my salad bowl. I take 1 or 2 spoonfuls of whole almond meal, or 2 spoonfuls of sliced whole almond, sprinkled over the fruit. And then I take a 1/2 cup of plain water poured over the almond meal or slices. I pour one whole cup of Lakewood Pure Pomegranate juice over the whole thing. That's it. Nothing else, /that means no salad dressing added/ or nothing less. // Except, when persimmon and apricot are not available, I substitute them with one whole nectarine sliced thin. // This is my favorite snack, or my favorite watering hole moisturizing recipe.

To make it a full meal I may add a quite a few other things such as, 6 soaked raw lotus seeds finely chopped (my penchant memory protecting recipe), 8 gingko nuts (my penchant lung tonic), a 1/2 inch slice of Korean ma (skin removed) chopped into small pieces, 5 small sweet Chinese chestnuts, 2 small Chinese dates, chopped and seeds removed, a few counts of almond tortilla, one full tablespoonful raw coconut nibs (my penchant recipe for heart protection), and for a meal I need a good amount of protein, for which I prefer some prepared fish for sushi like red shrimp and octopus slices. Good amount protein is important for me, for otherwise I get pain in the gums almost immediately after. I also know some mysterious sharp migraine headaches I tracked down to possible protein deficiencies. I'd recommend senior citizens who have history of frequent migraine headaches check into this possibility. When I have a large red leaf (whole or half) of Swiss chard, I chop it into small pieces and sprinkle them over the bowl or cooking pot. I love the color with the added nutrition. I also love to sprinkle 1/2 tsp each of Indian culinary herbal seasoning of the trio of turmeric, crushed fenugreek seeds, and red chili crushed, over my food over my pot before cooking, or over my bowl of salad. I never felt the need of adding salt even though I had bought a little bottle of "sea green salt" and had it ready. The fenugreek seeds may be helping in reducing itching on scalp.

APPENDIX A

Another Proof (?), that

The Nature May Take Care of Us
By Blessing Us When We Say,
We Have Enough Children, Now!

"A Natural Contraception," was the term the Chinese
Medicine Doctors at the Giangsu University in China,
(Who Called Themselves, "A New Medicine Group"),
have found and described it as such in the pages
of their 4 Volume Encyclopedia of Chinese Medicine.
(Alas! My own personal copy of it got destroyed while
kept in a flooded basement in storage.) Fortunately,
however, as luck would have it, I found the information
cited in my Korean equivalent copy of Eastern Medicine
published shortly thereafter, in October 1989.

And here it is:

Ilex cornuta leaves are harvested August through October, and after
removing small twigs and others, leave them in the sun to dry.

{Medicinal Qualities} Taste is bitter, character is cooling, and free of
any toxicity; Enters Liver, Heart, and Kidney Meridians. Caffeine,
saponin and bitter substances are contained.

{Medical Action I} When surgically removed pig's heart was treated with alcoholic extract of *Ilex cornuta,* its blood flow and contractile power increased.

{Medicinal Action II} When either alcohol or water, or similar extract of *Ilex Cornta* was injected into stomach of a [female] mouse, the rate of impregnation was all reduced.

My understanding of *Ilex cornuta* is an herb plant that is naturally distributed in Eastern China and Korea, that has been popularly used as a medicine over hundreds of years for the purposes of strengthening liver and kidneys, as well as promoting qi and blood, on the one hand, and reducing the pain on low back and knees, on the other.

It is my understanding, therefore, that this herb may be generally considered safe,
but I would advise you to consult your doctor first before considering this   herb.